"Hypothyroidism: The Beginners Guide"

How to stop surviving and start thriving

This book thanks everyone suffering from hypothyroidism and looking for answers. And for all the nutritionists, holistic health professionals and medical professionals who are making a difference in the field of nutrition and hypothyroidism. A lack of knowledge is a lack of power.

Your Personal Contract

I..

Declare that I will master my life in every aspect of it. I will no longer settle for less than I deserve. I have the courage, will power and wisdom to know that it's my time to make a difference in my life. I will put my best foot forward in all areas of my life. I will wake up grateful, put the right foods in my body for nourishment and uplift others.

I am the only person responsible for my life and I believe with every fiber of my being that that I can make a difference.

I am enough. I will be true to myself and follow my heart. My personal development is in my own hands AND I will stop fighting against myself. I will stop listening to self-doubt. My past experiences will not affect my current mindset. God will support me in with joyful abundance in all areas of my life. This book is only the beginning of my wonderful journey to happiness, joy, peace and prosperity. I am willing to go beyond my past and I am the only person who chooses my path and I don't need anyone's approval. I release all limitations from my past.

I will seek the highest truth and the most healing ways to live my life. Health and Happiness is abundantly mine.

Love,

Signed by ....

Chapter 1

Your Thyroid has a Mistress

Chapter 2

The journey Begins

Chapter 3

Change your habits, Change your life

Chapter 4

Medication

Chapter 5

Adopting a Hypothyroidism Diet

Disclaimer

The information and recipes contained in book are based upon the research and the personal experiences of the author. Every attempt has been made to provide accurate, up to date and reliable information. No warranties of any kind are expressed or implied. Readers acknowledge that the author is not engaging in the rendering of legal, financial, medical or professional advice. By reading this book, the reader agrees that under no circumstance the author is not responsible for any loss, direct or indirect, which are incurred by using this information contained within this book. Including but not limited to errors, omissions or inaccuracies. This book is not intended as replacements from what your health care provider has suggested. The author is not responsible for any adverse effects or consequences resulting from the use of any of the suggestions, preparations or procedures discussed in this book. All matters pertaining to your health should be supervised by a health care professional. I am not a doctor, or a medical professional. This book is designed for as an educational and entertainment tool only. Please always check with your health practitioner before changing your diet, taking any vitamins, supplements, or herbs, as they may have side-effects, especially when combined with medications, alcohol, or other vitamins or supplements. Please check with you health care provider to see if you can switch to a hypothyroidism diet whereas you might have other health conditions that will not allow you to. Knowledge is power, educate yourself and find the answer to your health care needs. Wisdom is a wonderful thing to seek. I hope this book will teach and encourage you to take leaps in your life to educate yourself for a happier & healthier life. You have to take ownership of your health. All rights reserved. No part of this publication may be reproduced, distributed, or transmitted in any form or by any means, including photo copying, or recording, or other electronic, or mechanical methods, without the prior written permission of the author, except in the case of brief quotations, embodied in critical reviews, in certain other noncommercial uses permitted by copyright laws. Although every precaution has been taken by the author to verify the accuracy of the information contained herein, the author assumes no responsibility for any errors, or omissions. No liability is assumed for damages that may result from the information that is obtained within.

A.L. Childers

Copyrighted Material

Copyright 2016 Audrey Childers.

This book, or parts thereof, may not be reproduced in any form without the written permission from the Author. All rights reserved. This book is copyright protected. You cannot sell, distribute, use, quote or paraphrase any part or the content within this book without of the author. Legal action will be pursued if breached.

All rights reserved. In accordance with the U.S. write copyright act of 1976, the scanning, the uploading, and electronic scanning of any part of this book. Without permission of the publisher or author constitutes unlawful piracy and theft of the author's intellectual property. If you would like to use material from this book. (Other than for review purposes), prior written permission must be obtained by contacting the author @ permissions @ audreychilders@hotmail.com. Thank you for your support of the author's rights.

Thanks for reading my latest book. Please let me know if you need any support with it.

This Book is dedicated to my three beautiful, distracting daughters who have allowed me to experience the kind of love that people truly die for. Katlyn, Abbigail and Caroline.

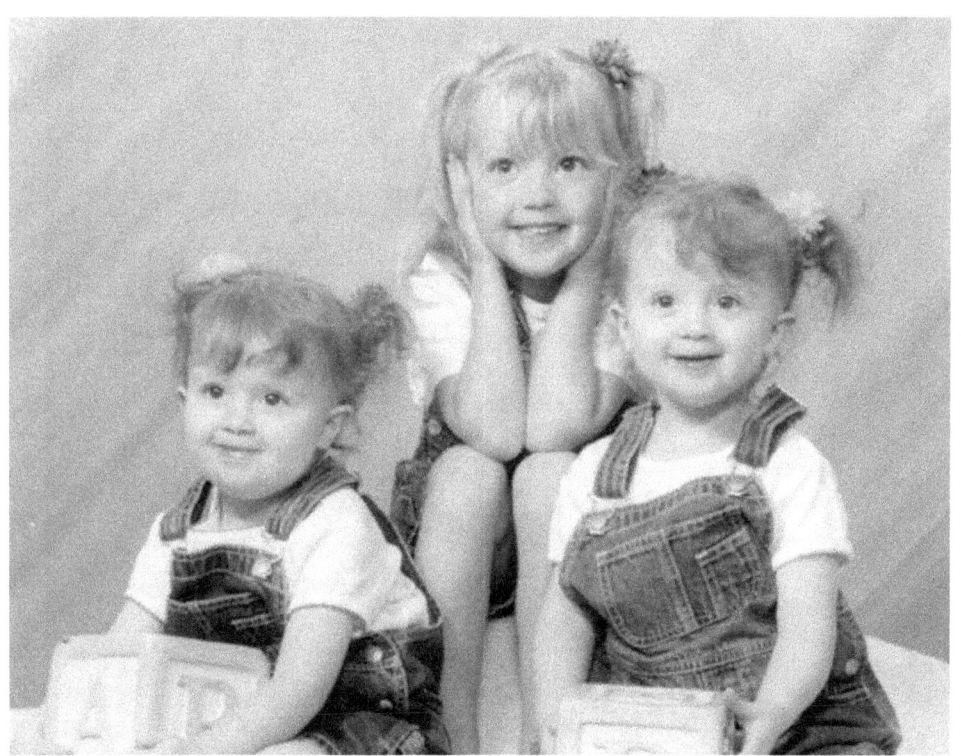

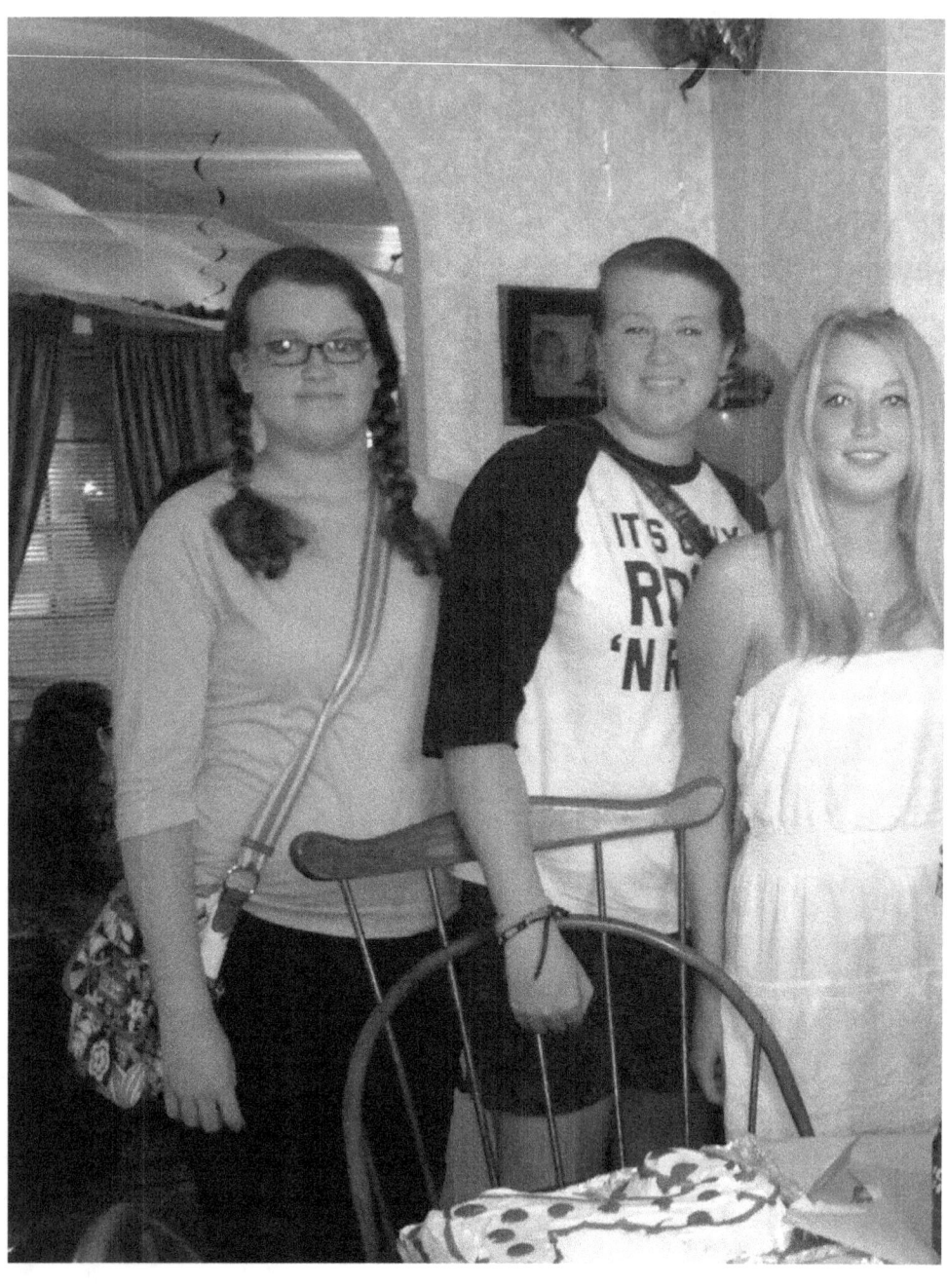

Introduction:

Around 20 million Americans and 250 million people worldwide will be affected by low thyroid function or hypothyroidism. One in 8 women will struggle with a thyroid problem in her lifetime, and up to 90% of all thyroid problems are autoimmune in nature, the most common of which is Hashimoto's. Many people don't know that hypothyroidism is an autoimmune disease and the reason why most doctors don't mention is because it's simple: it doesn't affect their treatment plan. Traditional medicine treats autoimmune disorders with steroids and other methods that suppress the immune system. The number of people suffering from hypothyroidism continues to rise each year. Levothyroxine is the 4th highest selling drug in the U.S. Every Cell in your body responds to your thyroid hormones. These hormones have a direct impact on every major system in your body.

Hypothyroidism is the kind of disease that carries a bit of mystery with it. This book is not for readers looking for quick answers. There is not one size fits all. You have to be in charge of your health. I didn't write this book to sell you any "snake oil" in a bottle. I've written this book to be an eye opener for you and to share with you what I have learned on my journey. The solutions in this book has helped so many people. There are many incredible holistic practitioners, authors and researchers with experience and expertise in this area. I've done my best to pull from all their expertise, as well as my own knowledge and clinical experience. I want to make it easy for you to find the answers quickly, all in the one place, because I'm all too familiar with that awful side effects of hypothyroidism. I certainly don't want you to have to spend years finding solutions, like I did. I also what you to understand that there isn't an easy "one pill" solution, but the "one pill" approach that our current medical system is using is NOT WORKING because the underlying cause for hypothyroidism is not being addressed. Many people never question their doctors, research their medications or find out the side effects of what was prescribed. Don't misconstrue what I am saying being on medication isn't a bad thing when it is necessary but sometimes the medications that are given will camouflage the real symptoms. The problem with giving people thyroid hormone is that it may not be addressing the root cause of your hypothyroidism. If you start addressing the root cause your body will start to heal itself. All these years of bad eating habits beginning in your childhood, a stressful life, lack of exercise/too much exercise, environmental toxins and little to no sleep have contributed to your hypothyroidism. So many of us have these crazy phantom-like health problems. The best patient to be is a well informed and an educated patient. This book can make the difference between you having the energy to live your life as you want, or merely dragging yourself through life. Don't be upset with your medical doctor or endocrinologist they are there to treat your illness not really to give advice on getting to the root of the cause. These doctors are needed. A Health Practitioner will get to the root of your cause and start helping you heal yourself from the main underlying issues. In this book, you will learn the link that ties many of our issues together. Get ready to go on a journey of discovery where you are going to learn how everything ties into one. The foods we eat can interfere with your thyroid medication. Our body is lacking certain nutrients that heavily influence the function of our thyroid gland while certain foods can inhibit your body's ability to absorb the replacement hormones. There is no one size fits all program when you are dealing with hypothyroidism. When you start to eat smarter and are aware of what foods feed your body, despite the condition, you can start to feel better and manage your symptoms. In this age of overly processed, genetically modified, artificially flavored and preservative loaded foods. I'm very excited that you bought this book and are wanting to find an answer to what is hindering your life. Think about this. Americans are in such a pathetic health crisis. We have the abundance of everything at our finger tips but yet we 1 in 3 people are on some sort of medication. It doesn't matter if it's Prescribed or over the counter. Meanwhile billions of people around the world are in better health than the average American, doesn't have to be on some sort of medication and are in their correct body mass index. We are in such a state of denial. My mission is to do everything in my power to help you to start healing and reach your fullest potential. To help be a source of inspiration you seek and attract what you desire with the faith that your vision of success is your destiny! You deserve to kick yourself out of that fat storage unhealthy mode and into a fat burning healthy mode. Remember, what we eat, governs what we become.

A note of caution:

I strongly support self-care, personal health empowerment and improving your understanding of thyroid health. However, this cannot substitute by a trained medical professional in cases of long standing and undiagnosed symptoms. This book is thus not meant as a substitute for professional medical judgement, though it can serve as a helpful adjunct to it.

When in doubt about your thyroid seek your doctor or your medical professional to exclude serious medical conditions.

Be safe, be sane and be healthy.

Get a complete exam from a reliable health practitioner. Do what you can do within the boundaries of good common sense.

In a word, be kind to yourself and your thyroid.

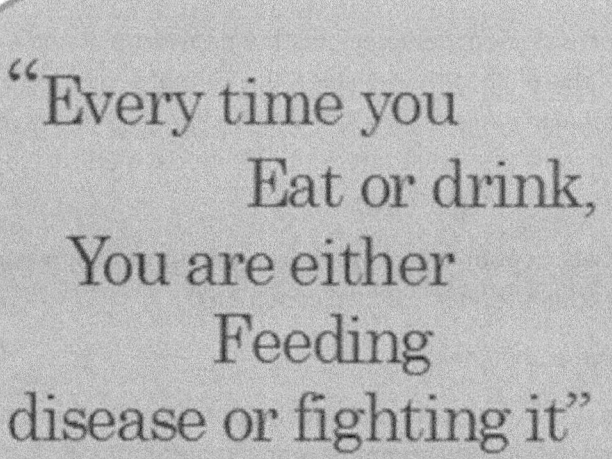

Message from the Author

After being diagnosed with hypothyroidism over 25 years ago. I knew there was something more than just being labeled with a medical condition. There wasn't a lot of information on how to heal myself from the inside out. You really must begin to understand that there really isn't a one size fits all diet for everyone who is has been diagnosed with Hypothyroidism but there are certain ways you can eat that will certainly help begin the healing process. Diet alone isn't enough to help your body start fighting this battle that is raging in your body. The food you eat is your first line of defense against hypothyroidism. You must start addressing other areas in your life.

My goal in this book is to help you understand and show you have easy it is for you to start cutting out the foods that don't nourish your body. Hypothyroidism is a very tricky condition and complicated disorder to manage. The foods we eat can interfere with your treatment. Our body is lacking certain nutrients that heavily influence the function of our thyroid gland while certain foods can inhibit your body's ability to absorb the replacement hormones. There is no one size fits all program when you are dealing with hypothyroidism. When you start to eat smarter and are aware of what foods feed your body, despite the condition, you can start to feel better and manage your symptoms. It is my immense pleasure to write another book on hypothyroidism. In this age of overly processed, genetically modified, artificially flavored and preservative loaded foods. It's no wonder that more people are wanting to eat a more wholesome and a more all natural diet. We are trying to find our way back to the basics. I hope this book encourages you and inspires you to seek out the truth and start healing your body from the inside out. All I can give you is the blueprint of things you can start doing today to incorporate a healthier you. I am living this way. I can talk about what has worked for me and share my knowledge with you. My mission is to do everything in my power to start to heal and reach your fullest potential. To help be a source of inspiration you seek and attract what you desire with the faith that your vision of success is your destiny!   You deserve to kick yourself out of that fat storage mode and into a fat burning mode. What we eat, governs what we become.

My new purpose is to empower people to embrace who they are, to add value to their life, to inspire them and to connect with those who are struggling with hypothyroidism. You need to realize that you have to invest in your health. You are worth investing money into yourself and take charge of your health. Will it "hurt" a little? Ha, you bet, but it will change your life.

I wish somebody had given me a step-by-step roadmap back when I was first diagnosed with hypothyroidism.

"They laugh at me because I'm different, I laugh at them because they're all the same". I love this quote, it's brutally honest. In a world full of #copycats I'm totally ok with going against the "norm". I've heard it all from : I'm crazy, irrational, I'll never succeed, Why don't I get a real job and on and on it goes. Yes I've had days were I'm like" WTF am I doing?" But then I'll get a text or email or phone call from a client or friend and its back to being Balls to the Wall crazy again. I am an expert at Thriving and Surviving!! Which is why I have compassion and a genuine Want to help others be the Very Best Them they can be. Life is what you make it. Be **BRAVE**... Be BOLD and above all else: Be an **Authentic YOU**. #realwomensucceed #insights #positivity #fitmom #motivation #champion #iwantyou #happinessjunkie #lifebydesign #familyfirst #quoteoftheday #cheerleader #smile #life #hypothyroidism #lifechanging

I love this statement by Mark Macdonald, co-ceo and co-founder of Appster

I believe that you should make a habit of believing in the things that people think are impossible. Learn to question everything. Experts will always try to convince you that what you want to do is impossible and simply won't work. However, every successful endeavor starts with one stubborn person who refuses to operate by the same rules and type of thinking that everyone else does.

Be that person.

About the Author:

Blogger, writer, health activist, health coach and investigative journalist. As a patient advocate and certified Holistic Health coach, Audrey Childers is raising the bar on thyroid care and helping others take back their lives from thyroid, autoimmune and inflammatory diseases. She founded Thehypothyroidismchick.com so that no one else would have to feel alone with these diseases—or spend their life savings and countless hours researching—like she did. Her mission is to help you enjoy the fruits of her painstaking efforts to resolve her own Hashimoto's Thyroiditis, with gentle, custom healing programs that nurture your body and get results. She is also a published author, blogger and health journalist. Where she talks about her experiences with hypothyroidism. You can find recipes that has worked for her and her personal spin on things we can do to heal our body naturally. She's been battling hypothyroidism for years. After many unsuccessful doctors' appointments over the years, it seemed none offered me ideas on diet change.

Please check out my other books on Amazon. My books were available also through Book a Million along with Barnes and Noble but due to only profiting .58 cents per book. I decided Amazon was the best way to sell my books.

Awareness has Magic: Creating a Healthy Hypothyroidism Mind, body and Spirit Home life

We must take a stand for our health. Your Thyroid hormones affect every organ in your body, every tissue and every single cell. You must start rebalancing the immune system by addressing the root cause of your hypothyroidism. Throughout this book, you will find useful, informative and easy to understand recipes for your mind, body and spirit. When I started writing this book, I wanted to introduce you to the idea of a cleaner less toxic world and for you to learn just how simply easy it is for you to start creating your own cleaning recipes throughout your home but this book has transformed into so much more than just a book full of all natural DIY recipes. This book will enlighten you and help you have a deeper understanding of not only why you should be more aware but how to be more aware. AWARENESS HAS MAGIC.

Kicking Hypothyroidism's booty, The Slow Cooker way: 101 Slow Cooker recipes!

I wanted to create a user-friendly handbook to help anyone affected by this disorder. I've seen many doctors over the years and none offered me ideas on diet change. I've included recipes, ideas on solutions for a healthier home, what you should be eating and shouldn't, how to shed those extra pounds, regain your self-confidence and vitality back into your life. I want you to feel strong, sexy, and beautiful. This is my heartfelt guide to you. Together, once again, you can start to gain that wonderful life that you deserve. I am a student in this thing called life. I want to be remembered as a pioneer who thought, imagined, and inspired. What we feel at times is the impossible or unthinkable. Life is a wonderful journey.

A Survivors Cookbook Guide to Kicking Hypothyroidism's booty.

Do you need foods that promote your thyroid health? Let's heal your body from the inside out. We've all heard that our gut is called the "second-brain". Given how closely the two interact with each other one thing you may not realize is your emotions and weight gain can start in the gut. Your gut and digestion can also cause you to hold onto that excess weight and just feel lousy. I've included 101 hypothyroidism fighting recipes that cook themselves. Our main concern is kicking hypothyroidism's booty. I hope this book inspires you to use your slow cooker more often and create your own new recipes. Let's together shed those extra pounds, regain your self-confidence and vitality back into your life.

Reset Your Thyroid, 21 day Meal plan Thyroid reboot

This is a 21-day Meal plan to reset your thyroid and jump start your weight loss journey. It is filled with 21 breakfast recipes, 21 lunch recipes and 21 dinner recipes. They are packed full of nutrients, healthy fats and proteins. All are easy to make and I've done all the thinking for you! All you have to do is prepare the foods and eat. It takes 21 days to form a new habit, it will most likely take that long for your mind and body to stop opposing your new lifestyle change. Three weeks really isn't a very long time. If you find yourself in a rut and coming up with excuses. You can regain control by reminding yourself that you only have to do it for 21 days. Motivate yourself to exercise. Choose something you honestly like to do and won't loathe at least 3 times a week. Create an exercise plan that seems easy to accomplish. (And, stick to it!) Give yourself a chance and commit to yourself to stay with the program for 21 days.

"There is only one major disease and that is malnutrition. All Ailments and afflictions to which we may fall heir are directly traceable to this major disease." –D.W. Cavanaugh, M.D., Cornell University

Got Hypothyroidism? Now What.

You're crazy and it's all in your head. Which I love to hear that one- said no one ever! There is nothing scarier than not knowing why you suffer from different health related issues. What really amazes me is how easily we go to a pill to fix what ails us. You know your body, you listen to your body and you can tell when something just isn't right. There are so many potential answers as to why you can be lacking energy, can't sleep, can't lose weight, low sex drive, anxiety, aches and pains in your joints, poor hair and nail quality, premature graying or balding, constipation or hard stools, feelings of sadness, anxiety , phobia's , extremely dry skin , cracked feet and even heart palpitations. So, you've been recently diagnosed with hypothyroidism. Everyone is different. I've experienced most of these symptoms myself. You need to start doing your homework. Break out that highlighter pen and paper. You will want to start taking notes from this book and reread it many times over until you can start absorbing all the information that has been laid out for you. This book will be your break through guide to getting your life back on track from book. It will help you start to breakthrough and figure out what you need to start addressing the underlying reasons to your hypothyroidism.

Remember Food is information. It's more than just calories.

You have to tailor your diet to your body's needs. Being on a very restrictive diet when you don't have to can put you at risk for adrenal fatigue and a nutrient deficiency. Nutrients give our bodies instructions about how to properly function.

Congratulations you are now become your own Clinical investigator.

Don't worry. Your head won't start spinning, I promise.

<u>Let's jump right in!</u>

1. Cut out gluten, dairy and soy.

   People have food sensitivities and are not aware

2. Start healing your gut- start taking a probiotic, digestive enzyme and drink bone broth

   Proper gut function is the key to a healthier body

3. Start addressing nutrient imbalances

   Check into seeing a Holistic functional Medicine Practioner-they address the underlying causes for your disorder

4. Eliminate environmental toxins

   This is household chemicals, shampoos, and tooth paste with fluoride, deodorant with aluminum, soaps and lotions these products can hijack your hormones.

5. High Stress- Your stress levels have an important impact on your hormones. You need to unwind. Stress weakens the body and makes you more vulnerable to infections.

6. Sleep- Not getting enough sleep can affect your hormones.

7. Caffeine- drinking too much caffeine will make your adrenals produce more hormones.

8. Exercise- you need to get that body moving. 30 minutes of day of anything as long as your being active. Just don't overdo it. You don't want to raise your cortisol levels.

9. Avoid plastic cups, bottles and bowls. - Bisphenol A, often known as BPA is a chemical found in hard plastics and the coatings of food and

drinks cans which can behave in a similar way to estrogen and other hormones in the human body.

10. Start supporting your adrenal glands- Your adrenals produce over 50 hormones that tell almost every bodily function what they need to be doing. These hormones affect every function, organ and tissue in the body. Eating refined foods and sugars will cause a spike in your blood sugar levels, which in return cause the body to release insulin and as a result the adrenal glands will release more cortisol. When you adrenal glands are compromised this puts your body in a catabolic state. Which means your body is breaking down. Since your thyroid glands controls the metabolic activity of the body, it will attempt to slow down the catabolic state by slowing down your metabolism.

You want to start adding **nutrient-dense foods** that are easy to digest and have healing qualities such as

- Coconut
- Olives
- Avocado
- Cruciferous vegetables (cauliflower, broccoli, Brussels sprouts, etc.) Cooked....
- Fatty fish (e.g., wild-caught salmon)
- Chicken and turkey
- Nuts, such as walnuts and almonds
- Seeds, such as pumpkin, chia and flax
- Kelp and seaweed
- Celtic or Himalayan sea salt

11. Eat real food—not processed foods

12. Try to eat as organically as possible.

13 If you're unable to eat organically, try to eat as naturally as possible.

14. Buy organic free range eggs

15. Use organic coconut oil- Did you know that coconut oil speeds up the metabolism and supports the production of the thyroid hormone, and kills candida yeast.

16. Try to eat only fish that has been caught in the wild, not farm raised

17. Estrogen Levels – Too much estrogen slows down your thyroid gland. Try to look for a more natural form of birth control other than birth control medications. You must start ot eat organic meats. The growth hormones in meats help lead your body to unbalanced hormones.

18. Cow's milk- Cow milk is very unhealthy for us. It often contains lots of estrogen. Try using nut milk.

19. Eliminate and discard all non-stick cookware

20. Try to eat more foods with L-Tyrosine - Tyrosine is a natural amino acid which helps the body produce its own thyroid hormone. Salmon, wild rice, white beans, eggs, pumpkin seeds, chicken and turkey breast.

21. L-Arginine - Arginine is known to help stimulate the thyroid gland. It also can improve immune function, improves fertility, and alleviates erectile dysfunction. Foods that are high in L-Arginine are seaweed, sunflower seeds, pumpkin seeds, peanuts, lentils, chickpeas, chicken and turkey and seafood.

22. Avoid all sources of fluoride - As I've already stressed throughout this book, fluoride suppresses the thyroid. Drink filtered water, avoid

all soft drinks, use fluoride-free toothpaste, use a shower filter, and throw away non-stick cookware. Avoid both coffee and tea which naturally has fluoride in it.

23. Eating an organic all natural diet is best - To help the body to heal itself, remove burdens on your immune system. This means that all processed foods, artificial flavors, colors, preservatives, white flour, white sugar, table salt, hydrogenated oils, aluminum and high fructose corn syrup need to be eliminated from your diet.

24. Chlorophyll - Chlorophyll provides your body with essential copper which helps to oxygenate the body, builds healthy red blood cells, and it overall assists with your skin being healthier.

25. Brazil nuts- many people with hypothyroidism are deficient in Zinc and Selenium. Studies have shown that a severe zinc or selenium deficiencies can cause decreased thyroid hormone levels. 2 Brazil nuts a day will give you your recommended dosage of selenium.

26. Coconut Oil: Buy organic, cold-pressed, coconut oil. Try to take 2 teaspoons of it each day. You can mix it in with your morning green tea or a smoothie. Coconut oil speeds up your metabolism, encourages production of the thyroid hormone, and kills candida yeast.

27. S.S.R.I. anti-depressant drugs- These drugs has fluoride as their main ingredient. S.S.R.I. drugs can be the root of nutritional deficiencies. They are toxic to your body and disrupt the serotonin that is used for digestion. Only 10% of an individual's serotonin is used by your brain, while about 80% of it is used by your digestive system. Healing your gut can solve many of your problems. Without your body being able to absorb the proper nutrients, your hypothyroidism will never be cured, because this nutrients are needed to balance the hormones and to strengthen your thyroid.

28. Sunlight- Get outside! 20 minutes of day. Let the sun hit your skin, face and forearms. Natural sunlight has many unique health benefits. 1. It allows your body to make vitamin D. Vitamin D helps regulate your immune system. 2. It cheers you up 3. Reduces heart disease 4. Sunlight kills bad bacteria. 5. Lowers blood pressure 6. Increase oxygen in the blood 7. Sunlight can help with easing the symptoms of depression.

Here are a few more quick tips to jump start your hypothyroidism health! Yes, if I repeat myself that is okay. It only means that its vital information and I want you to grasp the importance! Make sure your taking notes. Write all over this book. Highlight what you need to remember where it is easy for you to come back and access!

1. Adopt a Healthful Diet, Avoid Gluten

Your thyroid is depending on your to start feeding it and start maintaining your overall health. So stick with whole, natural, and organic foods. Steer clear of processed foods and eat gluten free. Gluten can have undesirable effects on the thyroid.

2. Avoid Soy

Soy products have hormone disrupting effects. Soy is also high in isoflavones (or goitrogens), which can damage your thyroid gland. Products containing soy protein appear in nearly every aisle of the supermarket. That's because soy doesn't just mean tofu. Traditional soy foods also include soymilk, soynuts and edamame (green soybeans), just to name a few. Food companies also develop new food products containing soy protein from veggie burgers to fortified pastas and cereals. READ your labels. Don't worry you still can eat fried brown rice but replace it with Coconut amino's instead.

3. Iodine

Iodine is a very popular hypothyroidism natural treatment source and many natural health experts do recommend a good source of iodine. While nascent iodine is most often recommended, Lugol's brand is a fine alternative. Dr. Group's iodine supplement, is also a viable option. Vitamins C and E, D3, selenium and zinc, and omega-3s should be supplemented with your choice of iodine as well.

Some food sources of iodine include:

- Seaweed and sea vegetables
- Some yogurts (organic yogurt, Greek)
- Cranberries
- Strawberries
- Dairy products
- Dulse flakes

Keep in mind that many hypothyroidism cases are actually caused by Hashimoto's thyroiditis. It was found in some research that increasing iodine intake could actually cause your thyroid issues to worsen if you have Hashimoto's. Instead, reducing iodine intake may be the solution.

4. Eat More Antioxidant-Rich Foods

Antioxidants are also important in keeping your thyroid healthy. But rather than getting them from traditional multivitamins, that simply exit the body just as easily as they entered, obtain them from natural food sources. Load up on vitamin C from dark green vegetables and citrus fruits, Omega 3 fats from walnuts and flax seeds, and zinc from pumpkin seeds.

5. Reduce Exposure to the Chemical PFOA (Found in Non-Stick Cookware)

Finally, reduce your exposure to PFOA, found in common household products including nonstick cookware and waterproof fabrics. Researchers have found that people with higher levels of PFOA (perfluorooctanoic acid) have a higher incidence of thyroid disease. Start cooking with cast iron skillets or stainless steel cookware.

6. Coconut Oil

Raw, Virgin Coconut oil has been used as just one hypothyroidism natural treatment. Coconut oil is made up of medium chain fatty acids known as medium chain triglyceride's (MCTs), which help with metabolism and weight loss, coconut oil can also raid basal body temperatures – all good news for people suffering from low thyroid function.

7. Natural Hormone Balancing

One approach to fixing thyroid issues and hypothyroidism is the use of hormone therapy. You really need to meet with a holistic expert. There are many great holistic and naturopath doctors. Most often, synthetic hormones like Synthroid, Levoxyl, or Levothroid are used, which contain only the T4 hormone and no T3 – two hormones produced by the thyroid gland. Thyroid conditions can be serious. You should always seek a professional who knows how to help you. Our organs and glands like your thyroid, adrenals, pituitary, ovaries, testicles and pancreas regulate most of your hormone production, and if your hormones become even slightly imbalanced it can cause some serious health issues. Our gut health can also play an important role in hormone regulation. Start loading up on up on rich sources of natural omega-3s like wild fish, flaxseed, chia seeds, walnuts and grass-fed animal products. People don't boost their omega-3 foods intake to balance out the elevated omega-6s they consumed. To many mega-6 foods will cause inflammation and lead to chronic disease. Eating more coconut oil, salmon, grass fed butt like Ghee and avocados will start to provide your body with essential fats that are fundamental building blocks for hormone production. Supplements like digestive enzymes, probiotics, bone broth, kefir, fermented vegetables, and high-fiber foods can start to repair your gut lining, which also can help to balance your hormones. Caffeine will rise your cortisol levels and then it lowers your thyroid hormone levels and basically creates havoc throughout your entire body. Replace your morning coffee with herbal teas. Matcha tea is a great caffeine replacement and is loaded with antioxidants, weight loss benefits, and cancer fighting properties, heart health, brain power, skin health and a good Chlorophyll Source. Last but not least GET OUT IN THE SUN! Free vitamin D, baby. 20 minutes a day is a great way to soak up some that free essential vitamin. On the days where you can't sit out in the sun you can supplement with a good D3 vitamin.

8. Foods that you should start incorporating in your everyday eating.

Figuring out how much you need to eat for you own unique body will require time and experimentation. Eat slowly and mindfully until you are 80% full. You want to feel satisfied but not stuffed. If you exercise more, you need more calorie intake. You can easily start with a salad and add more veggies, healthy, fats and proteins to any meal. You need to make sure you're getting enough nutrients per day. Try your best to not eat 3 hours prior to bedtime and after your last meal allow a 10 hour window before you eat again. A food things you can do to start naturally balancing your hormones in your kitchen is.

9. Beneficial bacteria supports your immune system

For most people, taking a quality probiotic supplement doesn't have any side effects other than higher energy and better digestive health. As a society we have drastically cut back on our consumption of vegetables and of beneficial essential fatty acids (flax, pumpkin, black current seed oil, dark green leafy vegetables, hemp, chia seeds, fish) such as those found in certain fish (including salmon, mackerel, and herring) and flaxseed. We are consumed with little fiber and an excess of sugar, salt, and processed foods. Stress, changes in the diet, contaminated food, chlorinated water, and numerous other factors can also alter the bacterial flora in the intestinal tract. When you treat the whole person instead of just treating a disease or symptom, an imbalance in the intestinal tract stands out like an elephant in the room. So to play it safe, I recommend taking a probiotic supplement every.

Probiotics are live bacteria and yeasts that are good for your health, especially your digestive system. Probiotics are often called "good" or "helpful" bacteria because they help keep your gut healthy. Probiotics foods include yogurt, kefir, Kimchi, Sour Pickles (brined in water and sea salt instead of vinegar) Pickle juice is rich in electrolytes, and has been shown to help relieve exercise-induced muscle cramps., Kombucha, kombucha tea ,Fermented meat, fish, and eggs.

Prebiotics foods are brown rice, oatmeal, flax, chia, asparagus, Raw Jerusalem artichokes, leeks, artichokes, garlic, carrots, peas, beans, onions, chicory, jicama, tomatoes, frozen bananas, cherries, apples, pears, oranges, strawberries, cranberries, kiwi, and berries are good sources. Nuts are also a prebiotic source.

The ideal pH for the colon is very slightly acidic, in the 6.7–6.9 range. When there is an imbalance or lack of beneficial bacteria in the colon, the pH is typically more alkaline, around 7.5 or higher. The optimal pH range for gas-producing organisms is slightly alkaline at 7.2–7.3.

When someone starts taking a probiotic or a prebiotic supplement (or eats a prebiotic food), the beneficial microorganisms begin to increase in number. These good bacteria start to ferment more soluble fiber into beneficial products like butyric acid, acetic acid, lactic acid, and propionic acid. These acids provide energy, improve mineral, vitamin, and fat absorption, and help prevent inflammation and cancer. The extra acid also starts to lower the pH in the colon.

10. Goitrogenic foods which if eaten in excess can affect your thyroid negatively.

They are commonly known as Goitrogenic foods, which means they contain substances which can prevent your thyroid from getting its necessary amount of iodine. If eaten in excess, they interfere with the healthy function of your thyroid gland, tilting you in the direction of being even more hypothyroid, or making you susceptible to having a goiter, or enlargement of your thyroid. If you look closely at the word itself, you can see the root word is goiter (goitro-gen).

Bok choy

Broccoli

Brussels sprouts

Cabbage

Cauliflower

Garden kress

Kale

Kohlrabi

Mustard

Mustard greens

Radishes

Rutabagas

Soy

Soy milk

Soybean oil

Soy lecithin

Soy anything

Tempeh

Tofu

Turnips

Also included in the goitrogen category, even if mildly, are:

Bamboo shoots

Millet

Peaches

Peanuts

Pears

Pine nuts

Radishes

Spinach

Strawberries

Sweet potatoes

11. Avoid Diet soda- diet soda is a chemical cocktail made up of artificial sweeteners like aspartame, saccharin, and sucralose. Artificial sweeteners trigger insulin, which sends your body into fat storage mode and leads to weight gain.

12. Avoid store brand Yogurt- Conventional yogurt usually comes from milk produced by cows that are confined and unable to graze in open pasture. They're usually fed GMO grains, not grass. As the yogurt ferments, chemical defoamers are sometimes added. Then high doses of artificial sweeteners, sugar, or high fructose corn syrup are sometimes added too. That's not all: colors, preservatives, and gut-harmful carrageenan can be dumped in. If you want to eat yogurt you can make your own or call the companies and ask them what is in their products.

13. Avoid High fructose corn syrup - read labels, stay away from any products that contain this, it is 20x sweeter than sugar and our bodies don't recognize HFCS. What happens when our bodies doesn't recognize something? It turns it into fat. It also confuses your body & doesn't let your brain know when your full! Please, Please I beg you don't start using fake sugars like aspartame or any of those brands. They are worse than HFCS!

Have you ever stopped to think what the underlying reason why you have hypothyroidism?

Many different underlying reasons can play a role. We do know that hypothyroidism is a chronic condition of an underactive thyroid and affects millions of Americans. Environmental chemicals and toxins, pesticides, BPA, thyroid endocrine disruptors, iodine imbalance, other medications, fluoride, overuse of soy products, cigarette smoking, and gluten intolerance. All of these play a very important role in your thyroid health. A nonprofit group called Beyond Pesticides warns that some 60 percent of pesticides used today have been shown to affect the thyroid gland's production of T3 and T4 hormones. Commercially available insecticides and fungicides have also been involved. Even dental x-rays have been linked to an increased risk of thyroid disorders.

Other causes:

Iodine deficiency

Hashimoto's Thyroiditis

Certain medications eg- lithium based mood stabilizers

Viral infection

Radiation therapy to the neck area

Radioactive iodine treatment

Thyroid surgery

Pituitary gland disorder

Hypothyroidism means what exactly?

Hypothyroidism means your thyroid is not making enough thyroid hormone. Your thyroid is a butterfly-shaped gland in the front of your throat. It makes the hormones that control the way your body uses energy. Basically, our thyroid hormone tells all the cells in our bodies how busy they should be. Our bodies will go into overdrive with too much thyroid hormone (hyperthyroidism) and our bodies slow down with too little thyroid hormone (hypothyroidism). The most common causes of hypothyroidism worldwide is dietary and environmental. The most common cause of hypothyroidism is dietary and environmental! What does that mean exactly? That means you need to be eat to cater to your thyroid and stop using all these harmful chemicals to clean your home with and put on your body! It's not hard. Yes, a little adjustment will be needed but isn't everything we do in life for the better of our health worth a little inconvenience until it becomes a habit?

Here are a list of symptoms that Hypothyroidism can cause:

Dry skin and brittle nails

Your fingertips becoming numb

Feeling fatigued, weak, or depressed

Constipation

Memory problems or having trouble thinking clearly

Heavy or irregular menstrual periods

Joint or muscle pain

Dry skin

Hair loss

Headaches

Unexplained weight gain

Thinning hair

Clammy palms

Difficulty swallowing

Sensation of lump in throat

Dry, itchy scalp

Diminished sex drive

Persistent cold sores, boils, or breakouts

Elevated levels of LDL (the "bad" cholesterol)

Heightened risk of heart disease

Heart Palpitations

Inability to lose weight

Inability to eat in the mornings

Tightness in throat; sore throat; horse sounding voice

If you always do what you always did, you will always get what you always got.

— Albert Einstein

Chapter 1
Your Thyroid has a Mistress

Your thyroid has been having a relationship with your adrenal gland. Your adrenals and your thyroid have a strange relationship. They contradict each other all the time. They have a topsy-turvy relationship in which when one goes up, the other goes down. Your thyroid has never been straight forward with your body and it never will be. That butterfly shaped gland in the front of you neck does more than control your metabolism. Your thyroid puts out hormones in your body that knock on every cell and tells it what to do basically but for some reason when you have hypothyroidism those cells refuse to answer the door.

Your adrenal gland is only the size of a walnut and are located on top of each of your kidneys. She is in charge of producing vital hormones that help regulate your body's functions which include two major important things in your life your sex hormones and your cortisol levels.

Your Cortisol is more than just a steroid hormone that is made in the cortex of the adrenal gland. It has a greater task than just being tagged as your fight or flight response system. Almost every cell in our body contains receptors for cortisol. When your stress levels are high cortisol is released into your blood stream. Also, having too much cortisol will make your midsection fat. Your body isn't designed for you to be in a constant state of emergency. Your adrenal gland doesn't know the difference between a true emergency and just being stressed out. So in return she will continue to produce extra cortisol into your blood stream. After a while of pumping out the constant need for cortisol she will become weakened and start decreasing her ability to produce cortisol and instead produce extra adrenaline. This is what makes us feel shaky, lightheaded and anxious. This can start leading our body towards adrenal fatigue syndrome. Cortisol is also released by two other major players in your body your hypothalamus in the brain and your pituitary gland.

Your hypothalamus job is to keep your body in a constant stable condition. It's like a supervisor that collects and combines information and puts changes in place to correct any imbalances. The hypothalamus also tells your pituitary gland how much hormones to release and store. Next what happens is your pituitary gland will produces the chemical messengers, also known as hormones that stimulate the adrenal gland to secrete who is in charge of producing vital hormones that help regulate your body's functions which include two major important things in your life your sex hormones and your cortisol levels.

The Million Dollar Question

Back to the million dollar question what does all this have to do with my thyroid? So, when the adrenal glands are weakened from one or more of the causes I discussed above, what happens is that it puts the body in a state of catabolism. What this means is that the body begins to break down, which as you can imagine isn't a good thing. As you probably know, the thyroid gland puts out hormones in your body that knock on every cell and tells it what to do basically. So when the body is in a state of catabolism, the thyroid gland will slow down in order to slow down the catabolic process.

The Light Bulb Moment

Is this all starting to make sense now? What we need to realize is in most cases, the malfunctioning thyroid gland isn't the actual cause of the problem. Other areas of the body are usually responsible for the thyroid condition. Many hypothyroid symptoms are very similar to adrenal fatigue that they are often confuse or misdiagnosed.

On top of all this confusion, the tests performed for thyroid and adrenal problems are often difficult to interpret correctly.

Why doesn't your medical doctor check to see if its adrenal fatigue instead of just labeling you with a thyroid condition? The main reason is because your medical doctors aren't trained in medical school to evaluate the entire endocrine system. They are trained to treat your symptoms with medication and surgery. Webster's online dictionary give this definition: a person who is skilled in the science of medicine: a person who is trained and licensed to treat sick and injured people. You should see an endocrinologist if you've been diagnosed with any thyroid disorder.

Endocrinologists have the training to diagnose and treat hormone imbalances and problems by helping to restore the normal balance of hormones in the body.

Why should you take a thyroid replacement pill when you really need actually have adrenal fatigue? This is where an endocrinologist can help. Hypothyroidism can also be by nutrient deficiencies and not your adrenal gland. This is why you should also look into seeing a Holistic medicine practitioner. They believe that the whole person is made up of interdependent parts and if one part is not working properly, all the other parts will be affected. In this way, if people have imbalances (physical, emotional, or spiritual) in their lives, it can negatively affect their overall health.

All is not lost!

I wanted you to understand or get an idea of how everything has a part to play in your body. Being diagnosed with hypothyroidism isn't just here take this pill and it will fix your issues. Hypothyroidism has a root cause. Once you start addressing the root of your problems then your body can start healing itself. Your body is an awesome design but there is a complex balance between everything. It's a domino effect. If you have something in your body that is overworked it will cause a major shift in your body. Don't worry the good news is it can be put in remission.

Food is not just calories it is information. It talks to your DNA and tells it what to do. Your most powerful tool to change your health is your fork. You can't go long periods without food. Your body always needs energy. If your blood sugar starts to drop this creates a stress reaction and now your adrenal glands will do what it needs to do to maintain your body's function by releasing more cortisol or adrenaline. Eating often will help put your body back in its normal cycle. You should eat foods that nourish your body and not hinder it.

Notes:

Author Note:

Let's not forget that we are all different. Each one of us are unique and we are biochemically individually wired and what works for one person may not work for another. We are extremely complex and each person should be valued independently. My reason for having hypothyroidism might not be your reason. Hypothyroidism isn't a 1 size fits all solution. I want to try to help you understand the many debilitating aspects of this medical condition. This book is packed full of repetitive information and is meant to be an eye opener for everyone who wants to make a difference in their lives and what some doctors just won't tell you. I want this book to be just one of your resources that is empowering to try to help you make sense of it all. We need our medical doctors, health practitioners and those who have studied years but I urge you to also find another doctor if your doctor won't listen to you or even allow you to see your lab results or even if you doctor refuses to perform necessary needed lab work.

You must realize that the thyroid has a relationship with all the hormones. It's a very complex balance and there is no straight forward treatment of just treating your thyroid alone. 1st you must make sure your adrenal glands are in total support. Adrenal fatigue is a very common amongst people with hypothyroidism. Next you have to get your cortisol levels stabilized. Having hypothyroidism your cortisol levels are already above average. Next finding the right medication for you. Everyone is different it isn't an easy one size fits all task.

Do you have Adrenal Fatigue?

A few ways that you know you have adrenal fatigue

1. You're a night person
2. Your blood pressure is about 120/80 or below 105/70
3. Your get a headache after exercising
4. You clinch or grind your teeth
5. You get dizzy upon standing
6. You crave salty foods
7. You perspire easy
8. You're always tired and you don't stay a sleep at night
9. You need to wear sunglasses

I was always tired, no matter how many hour of sleep I got each night. I had constant brain fog. I was always cold when others weren't. No matter what I did I couldn't shed the lbs. These issues go hand in hand with my diagnosis of hypothyroidism. After being prescribed my hypothyroidism medications I still was having problems. It wasn't getting any better. Many doctors over look adrenal fatigue since it is so similar in comparison with my hypothyroidism. The tests for thyroid and adrenal fatigue are often difficult to understand. The two are often confused or misdiagnosed. So, which one do you treat 1st? The chicken or the egg?

Adrenal Gland, Say What?

My adrenals and my thyroid have a strange relationship. They contradict each other all the time. They have a topsy-turvy relationship in which when one thing goes up, the other goes down. My adrenals are my "lifesaving" organs because they control my body's hormones and help me to survive in stressful situations. The adrenals act as the control organs for my "fight or flight" response and secrete many of our most important hormones including: pregnenolone, adrenaline, estrogen, progesterone, testosterone, DHEA and cortisol.

Adrenal fatigue is more often than none misunderstood as an autoimmune disorder. Adrenal fatigue can impersonate and look like other common illnesses and diseases. Adrenal fatigue can be caused by:

- Stressful experiences like death of loved one, divorce or surgery
- Exposure to environmental toxins and pollution
- Prolonged stress due to financial hardship, bad relationships or work environment, and other conditions that entail feelings of despair
- Negative thinking and emotional trauma
- Lack of sleep
- Poor diet and lack of exercise

Unknowingly my adrenals were constantly stressed which set off a chain reaction to my immune system and set up shop for inflammation through my entire body. The adrenal-hypothalamus-pituitary reaction circle controls the release of cortisol. All of my organs and my immunity were being impacted negatively by the resulting continuous hit of cortisol. Actually since my adrenals were out of whack it was causing my hypothyroidism to be much worse than it would be normally. Could this be the reason for my latest diagnosis of Hashimoto's? Could my weakened adrenal glands be the main reason why I developed a thyroid condition in the 1st place? My life was a chaotic world wind of craziness. I was going to school fulltime to be a nurse and just had my twins which added 3 kids under the age of three. Yes, I was exhausted mentally, physically and what was that thing called sleep? Years of poor eating habits and/or chronic stress had finally caught up with me. All those carb loaded, over processed, refined foods and sugars had also caused an imbalance in my insulin and cortisol hormones.

According to the Endocrine Society, adrenal fatigue is a myth promoted by health books and alternative medicine websites. "There are no scientific facts to support the theory that long-term mental, emotional, or physical stress drains the adrenal glands and causes many common symptoms," the society says on the Hormone Health Network website.

The constant abuse that I put on my adrenal glands from the bad eating choices and chronic stress lead to more secretion of cortisol which weaken my adrenal glands and lead to my adrenal fatigue.

Symptoms of adrenal fatigue are very similar to symptoms of hypothyroidism. People might experience all of these are just a few. Some of the more common ones:

- Extremely tired, especially in the morning
- Find it difficult to obtain quality sleep
- Crave sweet and salty foods
- Feel stressed out most of the time
- Decreased sex drive

What I've come to understand is in most cases, a malfunctioning thyroid gland isn't the actual cause of the problem. Hypothyroidism has a root cause. My goal was to figure out what was causing my weakened adrenals and to start addressing those issues. 1st I started to address what I ate. I added more things like:

- Olives
- Avocado
- Cooked Cruciferous vegetables (Limit this to no more than 2x per week)
- Fermented foods
- Fatty fish (e.g., wild-caught salmon trout, tuna and mackerel.)
- Chicken and Turkey (organic hormone & Antibiotic free)
- Grass Fed Beef
- leafy greens
- Nitrate free bacon
- Nuts, such as walnuts and almonds
- Seeds, such as pumpkin, chia and flax

- Coconut Flour, Almond Flour and hemp seeds
- Chia Seeds
- Kelp and seaweed
- Celtic or Himalayan sea salt
- Low carb fruits and vegetables
- coconut oil
- organic butter (preferably Grass fed)
- ghee
- Bone Broth
- Eggs: Look for pastured or omega-3 whole eggs. (if you don't have a food allergy)
- Cheese: Unprocessed cheese (cheddar, goat, cream, blue or mozzarella).
- Fish oil (EPA/DHA)
- Magnesium
- Vitamin B Complex
- Vitamin C
- Vitamin D3
- Zinc
- Ancient Nutrition- Bone Broth Collagen Loaded with Bone Broth Co-Factors

Notes:

Life is an experiment. Be kind to yourself. People really don't know what you are going through. Be patient, love yourself and step forward without judgement on those who have no clue. Reach for happiest with every breath you take. Trust your heart. Keep your faith and walk ahead!—Audrey Childers

Living in a toxic World

Many different underlying reasons can play a role. Everywhere we turn there is some sort of hormone changing chemicals. What can we do? Environmental chemicals and toxins, pesticides, BPA, thyroid endocrine disruptors, iodine imbalance, other medications, fluoride, overuse of soy products, cigarette smoking, and gluten intolerance. All of these play a very important role in your thyroid health. A nonprofit group called Beyond Pesticides warns that some 60 percent of pesticides used today have been shown to affect the thyroid gland's production of T3 and T4 hormones. Commercially available insecticides and fungicides have also been involved. Even dental x-rays have been linked to an increased risk of thyroid disorders.

Other causes:

Iodine deficiency

Hashimoto's Thyroiditis

Certain medications eg- lithium based mood stabilizers

Viral infection

Radiation therapy to the neck area

Radioactive iodine treatment

Thyroid surgery

Pituitary gland disorder

What happens when you combine fast food, toxic vaccines, flu shots, fluoride-loaded tap water, pesticides and dangerous, chemical-based prescription medications? Nobody really knows. There has never been a study on the effects of how combing all these things on a daily basis does to our body.

Why is our government allowing us to be weaken as a population? Why is our government allowing us to be systematically poisoned with our food? Hitler put fluoride in the water for the Jews to drink so they'd be weak and couldn't rebel. Yes, he surely did. That's the same chemical put in America's municipal taps today. It lowers IQ – as proven in multiple long-term research studies. Our school systems are even teaching distorted truths about what really happened in history. They eliminated critical thinking skills, discussions and essays, and replaced all testing with multiple choice, easy-to-grade, dumbed-down core curriculums. School food is 95 percent GMO, processed and toxic loaded preservatives and artificial ingredients. The CDC's mass inoculation scheme demands all children be injected with brain damaging neurotoxins (49 jabs by age 6) over and over, and now 1 in 68 kids have autism. There has been plenty of studies that have shown there are no connections between shots and autism but hasn't "these studies" in the past years later come to light that it was "tweaked" because someone was corrupt or paid off or it was learned to not allow us to start raising more questions?

The third major study in a matter of days to discredit the pharmaceutical industry, comes from the Journal of American Physicians and Surgeons, which found that giving children multiple vaccines at once is unsafe – a complete contradiction to the vaccine narrative shoved down everyone's throats by government, drug companies and the media for decades.

"Although CDC recommends polio, hepatitis B, diphtheria, tetanus, pertussis, rotavirus, Haemophilus influenzae type B, and pneumococcal vaccines for two-, four-, and six-month-old infants, this combination of eight vaccines administered during a single physician visit was never tested for safety in clinical trials," wrote medical researcher Neil Z. Miller.

"This is at odds with a CDC report which found that mixed exposures to chemical substances and other stress factors, including prescribed pharmaceuticals, may produce 'increased or unexpected deleterious health effects.'"

BAAM! Now what?

The definition of a medical doctor is a person who is skilled in the science of medicine: a person who is trained and licensed to treat sick and injured people. In this new age of technology why are these new skilled doctors not also being trained on how the connection between environment toxins, food chemicals and how they can have a direct effect on prescription drug chemicals? "Ties between doctors and Big Pharma are so extensive that it is almost impossible to find a large group of doctors who have no industry ties." I am not saying all doctors have ties to big pharma. My question is why has there been nearly 50 holistic doctors found Dead in a year span.

http://www.healthnutnews.com/recap-on-my-unintended-series-the-holistic-doctor-deaths/

Some food chemicals are more dangerous than the chemicals found in medications and vaccines. Aspartame and monosodium glutamate (MSG) are both genetically modified neurotoxins and should be classified as narcotics, but they're not. These food toxins cause brain fog, headaches, anxiety and depression, but MDs don't even mention them when prescribing dangerous SSRIs for anxiety and depression. Last week, a huge study published in The Lancet admitted that the risks of antidepressants in children and teens far outweigh the benefits, as the drugs routinely increase suicidal behavior. Out of 14 antidepressants, only one was shown to improve depression better than the placebo.

The biotech industry is trying to destroy ethical food companies like Chipotle. CDC investigation of Chipotle further supports corporate sabotage (bioterrorism) as likely source of E. coli contamination. But why? Why would someone go in and try to destroy a company like Chipotle is an ethical company with a pioneering vision of what clean fast food should look such as Chipotle? Why? Because Chipotle is an industry disruptor that threatens the waning dominance of the factory-processed, chemically formulated food giants like McDonald's and KFC. The GMO agri-giants that produce the low-grade ingredients sourced by McDonald's and other fast food giants aren't happy about Chipotle disrupting their "poison for profit" business model, and they've decided to play nasty (which is how the biotech industry operates by default). It's all about that bottom dollar.

Top damaging toxins to begin filtering out NOW!

Here's the "hit list" of that is a major game changer. Stop filtering them out now while you can still comprehend the difference between food and poison.

Fluoride in tap water: Look into a Big Berkey water filter – it's the best for your money, and filters fluoride, heavy metal toxins, chlorine, other people's medications, pathogens, etc.

Monosodium glutamate (MSG): Never eat this neurotoxic, brain-damaging, genetically modified and concentrated spicy salt substitute. Causes brain damage in infants and unbearable migraine headaches in children, teens and adults.

Aspartame, sucralose, sorbitol, saccharine, acesulfame potassium: These are all synthetic, IBS-causing, neurotoxic artificial sweeteners designed to make humans sick and fat.

Diacetyl: This synthetic artificial butter flavoring is often added to microwave popcorn. Able to cross the blood-brain barrier, this food additive nightmare causes beta-amyloid clumping associated with Alzheimer's disease. You may not see the word diacetyl, so just look for "artificial butter flavor" and you'll know.

Aluminum: Found in pots and pans, antacids, vaccines and flu shots, tap water, baking powder, deodorants and antiperspirants, and most food imported from China, whether organic or not. Causes Alzheimer's, Parkinson's and other dementia disorders. Aluminum fluoride is the compound often found in the brains of Alzheimer's patients.

Mercury, (listed as thimerosal), aluminum, formaldehyde and MSG: all very common ingredients in vaccines and flu shots.

GMO foods: These foods contain pesticides and herbicides that damage the human brain!

SSRIs – selective serotonin reuptake inhibitors: These dangerous, experimental, untested drugs block/disrupt your serotonin production and attempt to control it unnaturally. These drugs can lead to unnatural thoughts like homicide and suicide, and eventually, those acts themselves.

Let's not forget to mention the toxins in common candles, air fresheners, antibacterial sprays, flea-killing carpet bombs, junk food, canned soup & round up weed killer sprays.

Remember, you are what you eat.

Notes:

"Most people don't let their children smoke, yet they regularly take them to fast food restaurants and that's just as risky, in terms of cancer, as if they had bought them a pack of Marlborough cigarettes."
–B.A. Stoll

Notes:

What goes on your body, goes in your body

Did you know that it takes 26 seconds for the chemicals in personal body care products to enter into your bloodstream? Makeup is an essential beauty item used by women to help enhance one's personal appearance and self-esteem. Although you may be enhancing your own personal beauty but the chemicals in conventional makeup are often very harsh on the skin. If you want to protect your body from the harmful ingredients that are used in most commercial brands, you should check out organic skin care products and organic make-up. Start reading labels and asking questions.

Government regulations allow virtually any ingredient to be used in the manufacture of products that we use daily on our skin, hair, and nails, and in the water we drink. It only makes sense to start doing your own research.

The Food & Drug Administration (FDA) establishes the regulations and standards in the United States regarding the manufacture of drugs & food. The problem is that they do not pay as much attention to skin care and make-up as they should, thereby allowing some very harmful chemicals to be used in creating almost every product that is mass marketed.

The FDA doesn't regulate what ingredients go into makeup products or the labels that are placed on them. A lip gloss may be labeled "organic" or "all-natural," but it could just be a marketing ploy. Manufacturers know that there is a higher demand for natural products these days, so they'll do anything to convince consumers that what they're selling is indeed natural. Sometimes these products only contain about 10 percent "natural" ingredients with the rest are those nasty ingredients that are full of toxins – toxins that could be linked to cancer and Alzheimer's.

Have you taken the time to read or google what is in your personal body care products?

Some of the harmful ingredients that are used frequently in manufacturing the most common non-organic skin care and make-up items include:

- Mercury
- Dioxane
- Nitrosamines
- DEA
- Cyclomethicone
- Ammonium Laureth Sulfate
- Alcohol, Isopropyl (SD-40)
- Polyethylene Glycol
- Polyethylene eth-
- Emollients
- Humectants
- Emulsifiers
- Surfactants
- Preservatives
- formaldehyde

Author Note: Change your habits, change your life

The Hypothyroidism diet & lifestyle is a long-term health regimen designed not only to help you lose weight but also to enhance your health and energy. Most diets that you've tried might have worked for a short time and then you probably gained all of it back plus some. I want you to learn how changing you're eating habits first and get to the core of your hypothyroidism disorder will benefit you more in the long run. This is a one shoe fits all book. You will have set backs but every road to success is paved with some sort of failures. I believe that knowledge is power. **Most people don't understand the connection between diet, disease, medications and environmental toxins.** The main reason why I have been blogging and writing these books on Hypothyroidism is because we are so unaware of our bodies. No, I don't have a degree as a medical doctor but anyone can do the research like I have. In the age of technology that we live there is no reason why anyone isn't informed on any subject that they find interesting. You are more powerful than you realize. I want you to be moved. My heart will rejoices with you as I see you transcend stronger and become more enlightened on this journey that you were forced into. I have a vision of freedom for better health for humanity. I am leading the way to the road less traveled of infinite possibilities. You inspire me to become greater in myself and truly transformed my life to reach its highest potential.

	Home	Personal Care/ Beauty	Dietary/ Medicinal
Lemon Juice	· Clean glass & mirrors · Brighten your whites · Disinfect your cutting board · Brighten your toilet bowl	· Remove sun spots · High-light your hair · Reduce wrinkles · Shrink your pores	· Detox · Improve digestion · Sooth a sore throat · Strengthen immunity
Coconut Oil	· Polish wood furniture · Replace WD-40 · Remove shower scum	· Hair serum · Lip gloss · Deodorant · Prevent wrinkles	· Improve thyroid function · Reduce migraines
Apple Cider Vinegar	· Repel fleas · Clean your microwave · Deodorize laundry	· Sooth Sunburns · Wash your hair · Treat acne · Aftershave	· Weight-loss/Detox · Control high-blood pressure · Cure yeast infections · Prevent a cold
White Vinegar	· Polish Silver · Clean windows · Neutralize odors · Unclog your drain	· Cure an upset stomach · Sooth a bee sting · Condition your hair	· Tenderize meat · Boil better eggs · Eliminate garlic odor · Keep veggies fresh
Baking Soda	· Put out fires · Scrub toilets and tubs · Clean your oven or grill	· Deodorant · Toothpaste · Relieve diaper rash · Treat heartburn	· Leavening agent · Make fluffier omelets · Crispier chicken
Castile Soap	· All-purpose cleaner · Dish soap · Mop floors with it	· Body wash · Pet shampoo · Toothpaste · Prevent eczema	· Treat eczema and psoriasis · Cure acne
Castor Oil	· Discourage rodents · Lubricate kitchen scissors · Restore health of your plants	· Strengthen eyelashes · Relieve cracked heels · Soften cuticles	· Treat dry/itchy skin · Laxative · Induce labor · Relieve menstrual cramping

Notes:

Chapter 2
The Journey Begins

This is up to you. Once you decide that this isn't about losing weight. It's about being the healthiest you that you can be, you're ready for action and you will succeed. You really must begin to understand that there really isn't a one size fits all diet for everyone who is has been diagnosed with Hypothyroidism but there are certain ways you can eat that will certainly help begin the healing process. Diet alone isn't enough to help your body start fighting this battle that is raging in your body. The food you eat is your first line of defense against hypothyroidism. You must start addressing other areas in your life that can cause inflammation which are:

Dietary Allergies

Most people with hypothyroidism have gluten sensitives and by avoiding gluten it will start to reduce the antibodies in your body. This is a major player in your gut inflammation. Other common food allergens are Dairy, Soy, Sugar, Artificial Sweeteners, Corn, Peanuts, Eggs and Shellfish. You can have your doctor do a panel of blood work to see what food sensitives that you may have. Start avoiding any foods that will make your hypothyroidism worse. And next, you should put an effort into eating foods that will start healing your body. There are many great books that can help start your journey into eating better. **Remember Food is not just calories, it is information. It talks to your DNA and tells it what to do.**

Addressing Gut Health

Research over the past 20 years has revealed that gut health is critical to your overall health. An unhealthy gut contributes to a wide range of diseases including diabetes, obesity, rheumatoid arthritis, depression and chronic fatigue syndrome. Your gut imbalances add to the acceleration of inflammation in the body and drastically reduce your body's capability to absorb vital nutrients. We live in an age of antibiotics, refined carbs, processed foods, chronic stress and diets low in fermented fibers. Also did you know that babies who aren't breast-fed and are born to mothers with bad gut flora are more likely to develop unhealthy gut bacteria themselves? Hippocrates said over 2,000 years ago that" All diseases begins in the gut". You begin to start nourishing your but by adding a few things to your diet like bone broth, coconut oil, fermented vegetables, goats milk kefir, blueberries, yellow and orange foods and probiotics that have over 50 billion CFU's.

"More than 90% of the body's serotonin is produced in the gut, as well as about 50% of the body's dopamine."

Garden Of Life Dr. Formulated Probiotics Once Daily Women's, 30 Count

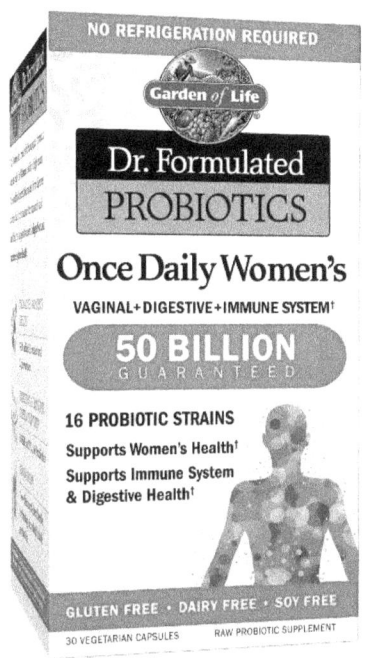

Why do I need to avoid Gluten?

Your thyroid is depending on your to start feeding it and start maintaining your overall health. So stick with whole, natural, and organic foods. Steer clear of processed foods and eat gluten free. Gluten can have undesirable effects on the thyroid. Don't make the mistake like I did when I 1st went gluten free and replaced my previous junk food with "GFJF" (gluten-free junk food), it's still bad and you still need to not eat it. It just isn't healthy. Why is gluten unhealthy you ask?

Gluten is a component of all barley, wheat, and rye products. It's a sticky protein that is found in all grains. This protein is very hard for your body to digest. Eating gluten can increase inflammation, which in turn disrupts function of the hypothalamic pituitary thyroid axis (HPTA). Disruption of the hypothalamic pituitary thyroid axis decreases conversion of T4 to T3, in return changing the absorption of thyroid hormones. Gluten is such a very misunderstood byproduct. When you have a gluten sensitivity the undigested proteins will float through your bloodstream creating an autoimmune reaction. Most of the grain crops in America and other countries have been genetically modified People have found that their thyroid function improves upon the removal of gluten from their diets. Some of the other of celiac disease and gluten sensitivity are:

Gas or bloating

Chronic constipation or diarrhea

Pain in the abdomen

A diagnosis of an autoimmune disease like lupus, asthma, rheumatoid arthritis

Unexplained joint or muscle pain

Fatigue

Depression or anxiety

Armenia

Avoid Soy

Soy products have hormone disrupting effects. Soy is also high in isoflavones (or goitrogens), which can damage your thyroid gland. Products containing soy protein appear in nearly every aisle of the supermarket. That's because soy doesn't just mean tofu. Traditional soyfoods also include soymilk, soynuts and edamame (green soybeans), just to name a few. Food companies also develop new food products containing soy protein from veggie burgers to fortified pastas and cereals. READ your labels. Dont worry you still can eat fried brown rice but replace it with Coconut amino's instead. Soy is estrogen mimicking, goitrogenic, hexane filled, protease inhibiting, GMO & a environmental destroying food."

Iodine

Iodine is such an important mineral for the health of your thyroid gland. It is needed for the production of T3 and T4, thyroid hormones critical in regulating your body's metabolism. Iodized salt and vegetables are common dietary sources, while iodine supplementation is a more reliable and exact method of acquiring dietary iodine. Iodine is a very popular hypothyroidism natural treatment source and many natural health experts do recommend a good source of iodine. While nascent iodine is most often recommended, Lugol's brand is a fine alternative. Dr. Group's iodine supplement, is also a viable option. Vitamins C and E, D3, selenium and zinc, and omega-3s should be supplemented with your choice of iodine as well.

Some food sources of iodine include:

- Seaweed and sea vegetables

- Some yogurts (organic yogurt, Greek)
- Cranberries
- Strawberries
- Dairy products
- Dulse flakes

Keep in mind that many hypothyroidism cases are actually caused by Hashimoto's thyroiditis. It was found in some research that increasing iodine intake could actually cause your thyroid issues to worsen if you have Hashimoto's. Instead, reducing iodine intake may be the solution.

Coconut Oil

Raw, Virgin Coconut oil has been used as just one hypothyroidism natural treatment. Coconut oil is made up of medium chain fatty acids known as medium chain triglycerides (MCTs), which help with metabolism and weight loss, coconut oil can also raid basal body temperatures – all good news for people suffering from low thyroid function.

All natural coconut oil cough drops

½ cup coconut oil, room temperature

1 teaspoon of freshly squeezed lemon juice

1 teaspoon of Ceylon Cinnamon

½ cup of Organic Honey

Blend coconut oil by itself for 5 minutes. Next add the other ingredients. Blend all ingredients 5 additional minutes. Scoop in a small silicon, bite size muffins. Freeze for 20 minutes. Pop out after 20 minutes. Place in a mason jar with a sealed lid. You can store these in the freezer or fridge until needed.

Beneficial Bacteria Supports your Immune System

For most people, taking a quality probiotic supplement doesn't have any side effects other than higher energy and better digestive health. As a society we have drastically cut back on our consumption of vegetables and of beneficial essential fatty acids (flax, pumpkin, black current seed oil, dark green leafy vegetables, hemp, chia seeds, fish) such as those found in certain fish (including salmon, mackerel, and herring) and flaxseed. We are consumed with little fiber and an excess of sugar, salt, and processed foods. Stress, changes in the diet, contaminated food, chlorinated water, and numerous other factors can also alter the bacterial flora in the intestinal tract. When you treat the whole person instead of just treating a disease or symptom, an imbalance in the intestinal tract stands out like an elephant in the room. So to play it safe, I recommend taking a probiotic supplement every.

Probiotics are live bacteria and yeasts that are good for your health, especially your digestive system. Probiotics are often called "good" or "helpful" bacteria because they help keep your gut healthy. Probiotics foods include yogurt, kefir, Kimchi, Sour Pickles (brined in water and sea salt instead of vinegar) Pickle juice is rich in electrolytes, and has been shown to help relieve exercise-induced muscle cramps., Kombucha, kombucha tea ,Fermented meat, fish, and eggs.

Prebiotics foods are brown rice, oatmeal, flax, chia, asparagus, Raw Jerusalem artichokes, leeks, artichokes, garlic, carrots, peas, beans, onions, chicory, jicama, tomatoes, frozen bananas, cherries, apples, pears, oranges, strawberries, cranberries, kiwi, and berries are good sources. Nuts are also a prebiotic source.

The ideal pH for the colon is very slightly acidic, in the 6.7–6.9 range. When there is an imbalance or lack of beneficial bacteria in the colon, the pH is typically more alkaline, around 7.5 or higher. The optimal pH range for gas-producing organisms is slightly alkaline at 7.2–7.3.

When someone starts taking a probiotic or a prebiotic supplement (or eats a prebiotic food), the beneficial microorganisms begin to increase in number. These good bacteria start to ferment more soluble fiber into beneficial products like butyric acid, acetic acid, lactic acid, and propionic acid. These acids provide energy, improve mineral, vitamin, and fat absorption, and help prevent inflammation and cancer. The extra acid also starts to lower the pH in the colon.

You gut is just one of the gateways to your health. If you have developed a leaky gut it means the tight junctions that usually hold the walls of your intestines together have become loose, allowing undigested food particles, microbes, toxins, and more to escape your gut and enter your bloodstream, causing a huge rise in inflammation that triggers or can even worsen any autoimmune condition. Don't fret you can start to heal your gut in a little as thirty days by incorporating a few easy steps in your life.

1. Say **goodbye** to inflammatory foods, toxins, and stress that damage your gut, as well as gut infections from yeast, parasites, or bacteria.

What do you need to do and how do I do start? **Eat more plant-based, whole, nutrient-dense foods. Garlic, leeks , Jamaica, asparagus, carrots, turmeric, fermented foods, Bananas, berries, artichokes, garlic, honey, organic apple cider vinegar, ginger root, aloe Vera juice, bell peppers, cucumbers, eggplant, tomatoes, coconut yogurt, bone broth.**

Cut out refined sugar and flour, processed junk and animal products. Start adding a variety of organic plant-based whole foods to your diet. These foods will start to fill your body with the vitamins, minerals, cancer-fighting phytochemicals, antioxidants, and fiber it needs to recover from chronic inflammation.

2. Say hello to good enzymes and acids necessary for proper digestion.

What do you need to do and how do I do start? Remove grains aka GLUTEN and legumes. Start eating pineapple and papaya. Our digestive system doesn't absorb food, it absorbs nutrients. If we don't have enough digestive enzymes, we can't break down our food—which means even if we are eating well, we aren't absorbing all that beneficial nutrition. Have you taken the time to glance at your poop? Here are a few signs that you might need to take a quality digestive enzyme supplement 30 minutes before a meal and make sure it doesn't contain products like gluten, dairy, etc. If it doesn't say "contains no: sugar, salt, wheat, gluten, soy, milk, egg, shellfish or preservatives then avoid them. Read labels! Make sure it has at least these three things in the supplement proteases (which break down proteins), lipases (which break down fats), and carbohydrase's (such as amylase, which break down carbohydrates).

If you have:

- Gas and bloating after meals
- The sensation that you have food sitting in your stomach (a rock in your gut)
- Feeling full after eating a few bites of food
- Undigested food in your stool*
- Floating stools (an occasional floating piece is fine, but if all your poop consistently floats, that might be a sign something is wrong)
- An "oil slick" in the toilet bowl (undigested fat)

3. Start taking a quality probiotic. By adding in good Bacteria back it will start supporting your immune system and allow your body is get back into balance and flush things out of our system.

Foods like raw garlic, turmeric, Fermented Foods, raw coconut oil, artichokes, onions, asparagus and leafy greens.

4. Fixing that unhappy belly by providing the nutrients and amino acids needed to start building a healthy gut lining. Most people simply do not understand how complex the human gastrointestinal system is, and contrary to popular belief, your gut isn't just a food processing and storage depot. Did you know that your gut has so much influence on your health is because it is home to roughly 100,000,000,000,000 (100 trillion) bacteria (approximately 3 pounds worth) that line your intestinal tract. Your gut is the home control center to your digestive system, your nervous system, as well as your immune system.

Here are two great products that I use. You can do your own research and I am sure there are other brands out there that are wonderful too.

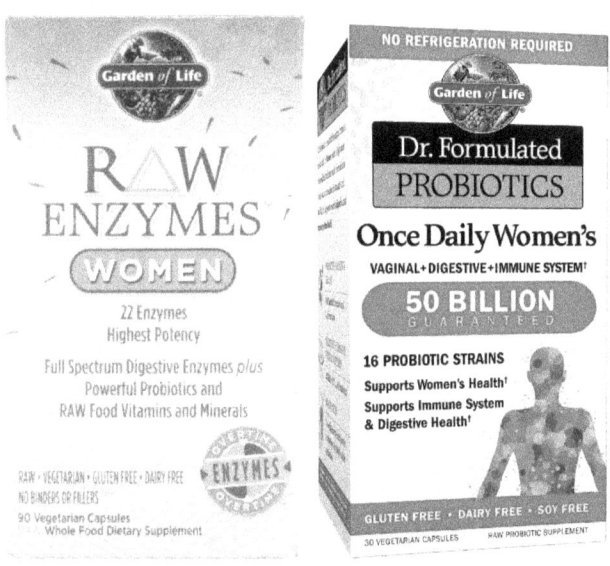

Notes:

So, are there things that are bad for your immune system?

Of course.

Your immune system does more than just fight invading bacteria. It is on a daily war on microbes and when it's not in line with your body it can contribute to disease. Sometimes the immune system falsely attacks its "self" tissue. This self-attack can cause many different symptoms like allergies, to something very devastating like the progressive degeneration of joints and organs associated with rheumatoid arthritis.

A disease in which the immune system attacks the body is called an autoimmune disorder. So, as I've stated before in this book hypothyroidism is an autoimmune disease.

Autoimmune disorders cause at least 80 different unnecessary conditions that can affect our bodies. This misdirected attack on self-tissue can aim an attack on one or several different parts in the body, depending on the disease that has been "created" or being "created". When you eat foods that you are intolerant or allergic too you are having your gut go to work to fight these invading and unwanted microbes. You even may be asking yourself if the immune system is such an efficient germ-killing machine, why do people get sick with the a common cold, flu, cancer or even other life-threatening illnesses?

Our immune system seems like it just can't keep up. It is constantly fight invading and unwanted microbes. Bacteria, parasites, and viruses are constantly adapting to new environments too.

We are feeding our body foods that we are allergic too like peanuts, shellfish, non-organic pasteurized cow's milk, commercial wheat, and soy.

Junk foods, processed foods, Food additives, foods that is made in a lab and foods produced with pesticides affects your immune system. These are also harmful and damaging on the nutrient content of the foods and can be to lining of your stomach.

Did you know that a common food additive called sulfites—can destroy the vitamin B content in foods to which they have been added.

What are in the shots that people so gladly take? Have you researched what is in that shot? Some shots have toxic metals in them and they are immunosuppressive. .

You must start giving your immune system a chance. Work on your eating better. Fermented foods, real foods, no processed mess, probiotics and digestive enzymes will help your digestive tract. Also, start eating adequate proteins and healthy fats, like I mentioned in this book to help provide your body with micronutrients and phytonutrients that will support a healthier immune system and reduce absorption of these invading allergens and toxins.

Fluoride blocks iodine receptors

Did you know that fluoride was Once Prescribed as an Anti-Thyroid Drug? Up through the 1950s, doctors in Europe and South America prescribed fluoride to reduce thyroid function in patients with over-active thyroids (hyperthyroidism). (Merck Index 1968). If you haven't already, you should invest in a water filtration system to rid your tap water of fluoride. Do we really know how safe tap water is? Look at the recent events in Flint Michigan! Can you really trust the water companies? Although fluoride concentrations in tap water are relatively low and are considered "safe" for human consumption, it is not.

Fluoride has long-term neurological and hormonal affects. Fluoride is not an essential nutrient. It is also that chemical that is commonly found in most toothpaste brands. There is clear evidence that, when ingested at high doses, fluoride causes neurotoxicity. Fluoride also is understood to interfere with the absorption of iodine, possibly leading to an iodine deficiency and ultimately hypothyroidism. To benefit your health, use fluoride free tooth or make your own tooth paste. Get a good water filtration system and purchase a filter for your shower head. We use a British Berkefeld.

Natural Tooth Paste Recipe

Natural Peppermint Toothpaste

1/2 cup coconut oil

3 Tablespoons of baking soda

15 drops of peppermint food grade essential oil

Melt to soften the coconut oil. Mix in other ingredients and stir well. Place your mixture into small glass jar. Allow it to cool completely. When ready to use just dip toothbrush in and scrape small amount onto bristles.

Homemade Coconut Oil Toothpaste Recipe

6 tbsp. coconut oil

6 tbsp. baking soda

15-20 drops of a food grade essential oil (peppermint, cinnamon, grapefruit or lemon taste great)

Melt to soften the coconut oil. Mix in other ingredients and stir well. Place your mixture into small glass jar. Allow it to cool completely. When ready to use just dip toothbrush in and scrape small amount onto bristles.

The Truth about the Good Fats

Healthy fats: If your diet is lacking in healthy fats, you may want to consider increasing your consumption. One of the best ways to ensure that you're getting enough fat in your diet is to eat more avocados. Avocados contain mostly monounsaturated fat and some polyunsaturated fat.

Avocados

Coconut oil

Dark chocolate

Eggs

Grass-fed butter

Nuts & Seeds

Eating more saturated fats also provides more benefits to those of us with hypothyroidism. Particularly, addition of unrefined, virgin coconut oil to the diet of individuals with hypothyroidism may: decrease brain fog, enhance cognitive performance, and boost overall physical energy. Coconut oil contains MCTs such as caprylic acid that modulate: blood sugar and metabolism, improve digestion, and reduce inflammatory responses.

Why should I Oil Pull?

Coconut Oil pulling can really transform your health. Your mouth is the home to millions of bacteria, fungi, viruses and other toxins, the oil acts like a cleanser, pulling out the nasties before they get a chance to spread throughout the body.

This frees up the immune system, reduces stress, curtails internal inflammation and aids well-being.

An ancient Ayurveda ritual dating back over 3,000 years, oil pulling involves placing a tablespoon of extra virgin organic cold pressed oil (I use coconut oil) into your mouth and then swishing it around for up to 20 minutes, minimum 5 minutes (pulling it between your teeth), before spitting it out. Whatever you do, do not swallow the oil as you will ingest the toxins you are trying to wipe out. Afterwards requires brushing your teeth with an all-natural fluoride-free toothpaste, and rinsing your mouth out. And you're done! It really is that easy.

Because coconut oil has been shown to:

- Balance Hormones
- Kill Candida
- Improve Digestion
- Moisturize Skin
- Reduce Cellulite
- Decrease Wrinkles and Age Spots
- Balance Blood Sugar and Improve Energy
- Improve Alzheimer's
- Increase HDL and Lower LDL Cholesterol

- Burn Fat

Goitrogenic foods which if eaten in excess can affect your thyroid in a negatively

They are commonly known as Goitrogenic foods, which means they contain substances which can prevent your thyroid from getting its necessary amount of iodine. If eaten in excess, they interfere with the healthy function of your thyroid gland, tilting you in the direction of being even more hypothyroid, or making you susceptible to having a goiter, or enlargement of your thyroid. If you look closely at the word itself, you can see the root word is goiter (goitro-gen).

Bok choy
broccoli
brussels sprouts
cabbage
cauliflower
garden kress
kale
kohlrabi
mustard
mustard greens
radishes
rutabagas
soy

soy milk

soybean oil

soy lecithin

soy anything

tempeh

tofu

turnips

Also included in the goitrogen category, even if mildly, are:

bamboo shoots

millet

peaches

peanuts

pears

pine nuts

radishes

spinach

strawberries

sweet potatoes

Notes:

Lifestyle of things to start changing:

Switch from iodized table salt to Himalayan sea salt, it has more minerals that help support better thyroid functioning.

Follow a gluten-free diet, which has also been shown to improve thyroid function. Research has found a link between wheat allergies and thyroid disease.

Practice stress reduction techniques such as meditation or deep-breathing. Chronic stress helps trigger hypothyroidism.

Avoid unnecessary body chemicals that are commonly found in items like antibacterial soap, deodorant, lotions, and makeup. These things are poisonous. Your skin is the largest organ in the body. Whatever you put on your skin goes into your body. I can't preach this enough. If you can't eat it, then don't apply it to your skin. I understand this might not be 100% doable but every little bit helps your body. My book **Awareness has Magic** is full of DIY nontoxic recipes for your mind, body and home.

Avoid chemicals like bromines, which is a common endocrine disruptor. Because bromide is also a halide, it competes for the same receptors that are used in the thyroid gland (among other places) to capture iodine. This will inhibit thyroid hormone production resulting in a low thyroid state. It's found in foods like mountain dew, plastic containers, non-organic foods-pesticide exposure, be found in personal care products, such as permanent waves, hair dyes, and textile dyes. Benzalkonium is used as a preservative in some cosmetics.

Supplement with probiotics, as good thyroid functioning depends on a supply of healthy gut bacteria.

Take a high quality whole-food multivitamin, and make sure you're getting enough iodine, B-vitamins, vitamin A, vitamin D, iron, omega-3 fatty acids, selenium, zinc and copper.

Limit exposure to fluoride and mercury — have a good water-filtration system for your home.

Follow an anti-inflammatory diet by eliminating processed foods and eating as many whole, organic foods as possible.

Take high-quality supplements, such as zinc, selenium, manganese, chromium, B vitamins, vitamin C, vitamin A and vitamin E (cod liver oil is a good source of natural vitamin A).

Exercise — this is especially important to correct thyroid function. Walking briskly for 30 minutes a day is a good place to start. A rebounder is a good form of exercise too. If you were to use it for 10 minutes a day it will stimulate your immune system and help cleans out toxin from the cells. It also has been proven to reverse the aging process and reduces your body fat; firms your legs, thighs, abdomen, arms, and hips; increases your agility; and improves your sense of balance.

Get some natural sunlight- unless you are allergic to the sun. 20 minutes of natural sunlight will give your body some needed dose of vitamin D. Sunlight promotes a healthy immune system, starts to alkaline your body and it gives you free vitamin d!

Tooth paste- stop using toothpaste with fluoride. So many other alternatives to brushing your teeth than using a fluoride toothpaste.

Avoid soy products-its mind boggling how soy has become this acceptable food source. Dr. Daniel states, "Thousands of studies link soy to malnutrition, digestive distress, immune-system breakdown, thyroid and hormonal dysfunction, cognitive decline, reproductive disorders and infertility--even cancer and heart disease."

Avoid artificial sweeteners and high fructose corn syrup- Artificial sweeteners are nothing but chemicals that were made in a lab by man. They are poisons and show never ever be consumed. They cause all kinds of health issues. Make sure you start reading you labels and avoid artificial sweeteners and high fructose corn syrup which seems to be in a lot of products. HFCS is a cheap ingredient and it makes us fat.

Find a homeopathic practitioner- One who will start working with finding the root cause to your illness? Everything has a beginning and then it is can be like a domino effect on the rest of your health. Homeopathy is a form of medical treatment that brings the body into balance and can start getting to the root of your problems to find a solution. A good homeopathy doctor doesn't treat your symptoms like most regular doctors do, they treat the whole person.

Notes:

Authors note: Armour medication has worked fine for me but that doesn't mean it will work fine for you. There are other Natural Desiccated Thyroid medications:

- Acella – NP Thyroid.
- Armour thyroid.
- Nature-Throid.
- WesThroid.
- WP Thyroid

Notes:

Did you know that Water Boosts Metabolism?

Many people don't realize the true importance of drinking enough water every single day and how it can impact both your health and your weight loss efforts. "Water's involved in every type of cellular process in your body, and when you're dehydrated, they all run less efficiently — and that includes your metabolism. Think of it like your car: if you have enough oil and gas, it will run more efficiently. It's the same with your body."

"Your metabolism is basically a series of chemical reactions that take place in your body," says Trent Nessler, PT, DPT, MPT, managing director of Baptist Sports Medicine in Nashville. "Staying hydrated keeps those chemical reactions moving smoothly." Being even 1% dehydrated can cause a significant drop in metabolism

Aim for at least 100 ounces a day – especially in the first couple of weeks until your body adjusts.

(Necessary internet disclaimer: there is such a thing as too much water so don't get silly about it)

To make it a little easier to calculate how much water to drink every day, here are the recommended amounts for a range of weights. Remember to adjust for your activity level.

Weight

Ounces of Water Daily

100 pounds 67 ounces

110 pounds 74 ounces

120 pounds 80 ounces

130 pounds 87 ounces

140 pounds 94 ounces

150 pounds 100 ounces

160 pounds 107 ounces

170 pounds 114 ounces

180 pounds 121 ounces

190 pounds 127 ounces

200 pounds 134 ounces

210 pounds 141 ounces

220 pounds 148 ounces

230 pounds 154 ounces

240 pounds 161 ounces

250 pounds 168 ounces

Signs your Thyroid may be out of Whack

Extreme fatigue. If you're always tired, even after sleeping 8 to 10 hours a night, it's a common sign that your thyroid hormone levels are low. Of course, fatigue and low energy are associated with many conditions, but if you don't have enough thyroid hormone (TH) flowing through your body, your muscles aren't receiving a signal to get up and get moving.

Brain fog. If it feels as though you're walking around in a fog all day, are having difficulty focusing, or forgetting things frequently, it could be that your thyroid is out of whack. Too much TH can make it hard to concentrate, while too little can cause memory problems.

Digestive issues. Those with hypothyroidism often complain of constipation, as an underactive thyroid can cause the digestive process to slow. An overactive thyroid gland can cause the opposite problem, such as diarrhea or more frequent bowel movements.

Mood problems. Mood swings, anxiety or depression can develop in those who have thyroid disorders. Anxiety and nervousness are linked to hyperthyroidism as the body is flooded constantly with a message to go, go, go, causing it to go into overdrive.

Do you exercise, eat right and still can't lose weight?

Putting on a few pounds can be caused by many different things, so few physicians will consider this alone as a symptom of a thyroid problem. But if you aren't eating any more than usual, exercise regularly and still can't seem to lose those extra pounds, it could very well be an underactive thyroid.

EVERY CELL IN YOUR BODY CAN BE IMPACTED BY THYROID MALFUNCTION

But... my thyroid test was normal (really?)

"Many people may be suffering from minute imbalances that have not yet resulted in abnormal blood tests. If we included people with low-grade hypothyroidism whose blood tests are normal, the frequency of hypothyroidism would no doubt exceed 10 percent of the population.

"What is of special concern, though, is that many people whose test results are dismissed as normal could continue to have symptoms of an underactive thyroid. Their moods, emotions, and overall well-being are affected by this imbalance, yet they are not receiving the care they need to get to the root of their problems.

"Even if the TSH level is in the lower segment of normal range, a person may still be suffering from low-grade hypothyroidism." — Arem, Ridha M.D., The Thyroid Solution, 1999, 2007 revised edition.

Other signs that your thyroid is in trouble (Do you have more than 3 of these?)

- Fluid retention/swelling
- Frequent viral infections
- Hair loss
- Frequent bruising
- PMS
- Ringing in the ears
- Sensitivity to cold/heat
- Cold hands and feet
- Insomnia

- Irritability
- Itchiness
- Joint aches
- Brittle nails
- Tingling in hands and feet
- Lack of concentration
- Constipation
- Depressed immunity
- Dizziness
- Headaches/migraines
- Hoarse voice

How does diet interfere with thyroid function?

It is thought that diet plays a role in thyroid health. Although low iodine intake leads to low thyroid function, table salt does not appear to be the best option. Many foods eaten in Western culture contain what are known as goitrogens or iodine blockers. Two popular goitrogens are soybeans and peanuts.

Notes:

Your morning coffee, Hypothyroidism and your Health

Nothing like that waking up to the smell of coffee. Its gets the juices flowing with that very 1st sip. Its offer you an energetic boost and mental clarity on a feeling that life can go on.

The thyroid gland is such a very important part of the body's regulatory mechanisms; thyroid problems can affect everything in the body from our temperature to appetite to the pulse. Caffeine, a stimulant found in coffee, can affect the thyroid in a number of ways and has an effect on your central nervous system, your digestive tract, and your metabolism.

According to the recent article, in new study from the journal Thyroid people who consume coffee at the time of taking their thyroid medication, we see a 25-57% drop in T4, one of the thyroid hormones, compared to non-coffee drinkers. This adverse effect persists for up to one hour.

Researchers have also found that for patients taking levothyroxine tablets, absorption is affected by drinking coffee and espresso within an hour of taking the thyroid drugs.

According to "Coffee and Health," by Gerard Debry, in experiments on rats, very high doses of caffeine caused the thyroid gland to enlarge, but at doses of about 300 mg, caffeine in humans did not change levels of thyroid hormones.

What about the benefits? Yes, there are many reliable studies that say coffee is full of antioxidants and polyphenols. However, these same antioxidants and polyphenols can also be found abundantly in many fruits and vegetables.

There are many other reliable studies that show coffee can play a role in the prevention of cancer, diabetes, depression, cirrhosis of the liver, gallstones, etc.

Many coffee drinkers report feeling good for the first two hours (mainly due to a dopamine spike).

(If you just can't give up that morning cup of Joe recommendations by researchers are clear: wait at least sixty minutes after taking levothyroxine before drinking coffee.)

What about decaf you ask?

Many manufacturers use a chemical process to remove caffeine from the coffee beans. The result is less caffeine, but more chemicals. It is the caffeine in the coffee that has the health benefits. Without it, you are left with little benefit.

Increases blood sugar levels

According to this study, caffeine increases blood sugar levels. This is especially dangerous for people with hypoglycemia (or low sugar levels) who feel jittery, shaky, moody and unfocused when hungry. Blood sugar fluctuations cause cortisol spikes, which not only exhaust the adrenals, but also deregulate the immune system. This is highly undesirable for those of us with adrenal fatigue, Hashimoto's or Graves' disease. Such cortisol spikes are also highly inflammatory.

Creates Sugar and Carbohydrate Cravings

As the result of the above, when our blood sugar levels come down, we need an emergency fix to bring them back up. This is why people who drink coffee at breakfast or indulge in sugary and processed breakfasts crave carbs and sugar by 11am or later in the day.

Contributes to acid reflux and damages gut lining

Coffee stimulates the release of gastrin, the main gastric hormone, which speeds up intestinal transit time. Coffee can also stimulate the release of bile (which is why some people run to the bathroom soon after drinking coffee) and digestive enzymes.

In a person with a healthy digestion, this is not a big deal. However, for people with autoimmune conditions, compromised digestion (such as IBS, or "leaky gut"), this can cause further digestive damage to the intestinal lining (source).

Exhausts the adrenals

Coffee stimulates the adrenals to release more cortisol, our stress hormone; this is partly why we experience a wonderful but temporary and unsustainable burst of energy.

What many of us don't realize is that our tired adrenals are often the cause of unexplained weight gain, sleeping problems, feeling emotionally fragile, depression and fatigue. Drinking coffee while experiencing adrenal fatigue is only adding fuel to the fire.

Gluten-Cross Reactive Foods

50% of people with gluten sensitivities also experience cross reactivity with other foods, including casein in milk products, corn, coffee, and almost all grains, because their protein structures are similar. Cyrex Labs provides a test for gluten cross-reactive foods.

Many people report having a similar reaction to coffee as they do to gluten.

Impacts the conversion of T4 to T3 thyroid hormones

Coffee impacts the absorption of levothyroxine (the synthetic thyroid hormone); this is why thyroid patients need to take their hormone replacement pill at **least an hour before drinking coffee.**

The indirect but important point is that coffee contributes to estrogen dominance, cited above, and estrogen dominance inhibits T4 to T3 conversion.

Highly Inflammatory

Any functional or integrative doctor would say the majority of modern diseases are caused by inflammation – a smoldering and invisible fire found on a cellular level.

This study found that caffeine is a significant contributor to oxidative stress and inflammation in the body. Chronic body pains and aches, fatigue, skin problems, diabetes and autoimmune conditions are just some of the conditions related to inflammation.

Can cause insomnia and poor sleep

This study showed that 400mg of "caffeine taken 6 hours before bedtime has important disruptive [sleep] effects."

There are healthier alternatives to drinking coffee.

Matcha Green Tea Powder

This is a great alternative to coffee. It has caffeine to give you a gentle jolt to wake up, but the caffeine content is nowhere as high as that of coffee, so you won't experience a midday crash and fatigue your adrenals over time. One cup of this wonder tea can keep you going for most of the day.

Natural hypothyroidism Energy Smoothie Recipe

Each ingredient in this smoothie provides necessary nutrients to kick start your day.

- Celery: full of calcium, sodium, copper, magnesium, iron, zinc, potassium. It contains fatty acids and vitamins including vitamin A, C, E, D, B6, B12 and vitamin K as well as thiamine, riboflavin, folic acid and fiber.

- Cucumber: with all its vitamin K, B vitamins, copper, potassium, vitamin C, and manganese, it can help you to avoid nutrient deficiencies that are widespread among those eating a typical American diet.2

- Avocado: full of vitamin K, folate, vitamin C, potassium, vitamin B5, vitamin B6, vitamin E, small amounts of magnesium, manganese, copper, iron, zinc, phosphorous, vitamin A, B1 (thiamine), B2 (riboflavin) and B3 (niacin).

- Romaine: dietary fiber, manganese, potassium, biotin, vitamin B1, copper, iron, and vitamin C. It is also a good source of vitamin B2, omega-3 fatty acids, vitamin B6, phosphorus, chromium, magnesium, calcium, and pantothenic acid.

- Chia seeds: contain lots of fiber, protein, fat: 9 grams (5 of which are Omega-3s), calcium, manganese, magnesium, phosphorus, they also contain a decent amount of zinc, vitamin B3 (niacin), potassium, vitamin B1 (thiamine) and vitamin B2.
- Coconut oil: where do the benefits stop? Check out our full article on the benefits of coconut oil.
- Matcha: adds a boost of slow-releasing, steady caffeine and is packed with antioxidants including the powerful EGCg, fiber, chlorophyll and vitamins. It also provides vitamin C, selenium, chromium, zinc and magnesium.

1 stalk of celery

½ cucumber

½ avocado

1 cup of romaine

1 tablespoon of chia seed

1 tablespoon of coconut oil

1 teaspoon of matcha tea

1.5 cups of unsweetened Almond Milk

Blend and enjoy!

Tazo Organic Chai

This Indian tea is rich in antioxidants and contains a plethora of spices including cardamom, cinnamon, pepper, and ginger that is sure to awaken all your senses in the morning. The smooth creamy flavor actually makes you feel like you are sipping a cup of coffee, but without all the extra caffeine.

Warm Water with Lemon

This is a great way to rehydrate and alkalinize your body and perk up after sleep. It also detoxifies the liver and helps get your bowels going. This really should be the first thing everyone sips in the morning.

Garden of Life RAW Organic Protein Vanilla

Who doesn't enjoy a yummy protein smoothie? It is a terrific way to load up with energy and nutrition. Use almond, soy, or coconut milks and your choice of a good quality protein powder. Throw in some bananas and berries which add heaps of extra minerals, vitamins, and antioxidants that are sure to fill you up and get you going for the grueling day ahead.

Vita Coco Coconut Water

Coconut water is Mother Nature's perfect drink. It has an abundance of electrolytes and minerals while being low in fat and sugar. This is the best alternative to an energy or sports drink, and can really give you a burst of energy in the morning.

Quinoa Milk

Suzie's Quinoa Milk - Vanilla

 This protein-rich natural energy drink may soon make its way into the stores…be prepared almond and soy and coconut milks…it's the next big health thing! Quinoa (pronounced keen-WAH), is a gluten-free, alkaline-forming, high-protein grain that has tremendous health benefits. Click on this link to read more of the healthy benefits!

Quinoa milk can be made from scratch, at home.

Consumers of quinoa milk do not need acreage or a cow to make this refreshment. The ingredients necessary to create quinoa milk can be purchased at a local health food store. The recipe is simple and cost, affordable. Here's a recipe from OmNomNally.com:

Ingredients

1 cup quinoa grain

2 cups + 5 – 6 cups water

1 tsp vanilla extract

1 tsp ground cinnamon

Instructions

Soak quinoa overnight in water and drain on the day of cooking or rinse quinoa in a mesh strainer under running water to remove the bitter saponins. Cook 1 cup of quinoa with 2 cups of water. Add cooked quinoa to blender with 2 cups of water. Blend on high until smooth. Add water to the desired consistency, blending the mixture after each addition. Up to 6 cups total of water may be needed for the consistency of store-bought non-dairy milks. Add vanilla extract and cinnamon and agave if using. Pour milk into nut milk bag, hold over a bowl or large jug. Massage contents until all liquid has passed through the material – leaving only the 'pulp' behind

Kombucha Tea

Yogi Tea Green Tea Kombucha Organic - You've probably heard about this one but don't know too much about it. Kombucha is a type of yeast. When you ferment it with tea, sugar, and other flavors or ingredients you make Kombucha tea. While the benefits of Kombucha are debated, many claim that it is useful for treating memory loss, regulating bowel movements, preventing cancer, helping with high blood pressure, and more.

Guayaki Yerba Mate Organic Tea

Yerba mate is the good alternative to coffee for those who can't start the day without a cup o' caffeine. Providing the same buzz that coffee gives, Yerba Mate is preferred by many as it's packed with nutrients, too. Mate is made from the naturally caffeinated leaves of the celebrated South American rainforest holly tree. It is widely known for not having the heavy "crash" that coffee can bring. Another benefit of Yerba Mate is that it can be prepared and consumed in a variety of ways—hot, cold, with honey, in a tea infuser, in a French press, or even in a traditional coffee machine.

Sparkling Water

Sparkling water can be a refreshing alternative to both coffee and water. Especially when flavored with natural, sugar-free, fruit extracts, sparkling water is delicious and hydrating.

Hot Apple Cider

Hot apple cider's sweet tanginess offers its own unique pick-me-up in lieu of caffeine, and its soothing warmth is just as satisfying as that of coffee on a cold fall or winter morning.

Turmeric Tea

Turmeric is highly anti-inflammatory, and this golden turmeric tea recipe is sure to help heal your body from a number of inflammatory health conditions. Turmeric can help detoxify the liver and protect cell damage caused due to environmental pollutants, attack from free radicals. Research has found that turmeric extracts can lower blood cholesterol levels – especially LDL 'bad' cholesterol. It has lipid lowering properties. This can reduce cholesterol levels and benefit weight loss by reducing adipose tissue weight gain.

This rich creamy and lightly sweet beverage is something you're sure to enjoy!

Turmeric Tea Recipe

- 1 cup coconut milk
- 1 cup water
- 1 tbsp. ghee
- 1 tbsp. honey
- 1 tsp Turmeric (powder or grated root)

Directions:

1. Pour coconut milk and water into the saucepan and warm for 2 minutes

2. Add in butter, raw honey and turmeric powder for another 2 minutes

3. Stir and pour into glasses.

You have to exercise caution when combining it with medications or supplements taken to slow down blood clotting. Turmeric supplements must be stopped two weeks prior to a surgery.

It must not be consumed by diabetic patients, those with gallbladder problems and pregnant and breastfeeding women. Always consult your doctor about the right dosage to consume for a specific medical condition

Notes:

Health is a state of complete physical, mental and social well-being, and not merely the absence of disease and infirmity.

--World Health Organization

Chapter 3

Cultivating a healthy mindset

You know that healthy habits make sense, but did you ever stop to think why you practice them?

I've heard women, in particular, say this a lot lately. They say, "Why can't I look like that?!" I will never look like that!"

Why do we mentally sabotage ourselves? Let's get something clear. You are unique. You are not meant to be me & I am not meant to be you. We are on this planet as individuals, each of us has a unique finger print that can't and won't ever be duplicated with any other human being. Ever! So why do you mentally sabotage your mindset with self-doubt and in return it starts a domino effect on your health? You are telling your subconscious without even realizing it that you are not made for greater things. You are telling your subconscious that you cannot be sexy, be brilliant and be fantastic. Be happy in your skin.

Everywhere you look — on every billboard, on every social media channel — it seems that there are beautiful, scantily clad women. So it is pushed down our throats that beauty starts from the outside but actually its starts on the inside and radiates outward.

Here's the thing: if you treat your body like it's your worst enemy – or not take ownership of your physical wellbeing – you are repelling good health. You're keeping yourself from being the best you can be in your life, because you dislike your body so much.

You're basically saying, "I dislike good health. I want to be rid of it."

Well, wish granted!

Good nutrition is an important part of leading a healthy lifestyle

You're meant to make a difference in this world; that's why you're here. But you must believe you're meant for greater things, so you can actually enter a place of mental stability, and eventually, a place of fantastic health. Don't take yourself out of the game by ignoring your bad relationship with your health.

Here are three common ways that we keep Ourselves Sick. Luckily, you can fix them.

Improve your relationship your health

When you decide to improve your relationship with your health, be prepared for people to question and criticize you. Change can be a very difficult thing for many of us to handle. You have the mindset, to step out on faith to get the perfect health that you really wish to have. It could be from grabbing that apple instead of those chips, walking 10 minutes per day, or reading a self-help book.

Take Action: Let yourself out of that unhealthy , fast-food, over processed and artificially filled food habit because it's ruining your life.   The only way to create a different outcome is to allow yourself to forgive what's happened in the past. The past does not have to be your future. You are 100% capable of changing your future health story, so do it.

You never step outside your box.

"I can't afford eat better."

"I don't want to spend the money on a new diet book."

"I wish, someone would just give me the magic pill for my ideal body!"

"I don't want to purchase another program that isn't going to work."

Does any of this sound familiar? The more you focus on what you don't have, the less likely it is that you'll ever have it.

Take Action: Focus on what you do have right now. Express gratitude for literally being alive. Now, you have to create a strategy to have what you really want. Set a goal, writing down realistic goals and make yourself a deadline. Take steps to get there. (And don't quit if it doesn't work the very first try.)

Or... you can keep focusing on what you lack. Call me in a year and tell me how that's working out for you.

You think health is something you're granted with, rather than invest.

You want your health to work for you, so you have to think of everything you eat as an investment. Will eating that cheeseburger build or create that healthy body? Probably not.

Will investing in self-improvement books or a mentorship program? Perhaps, if you do the work and commit to changing old habits.

Take Action: When you're about to improve your health, think carefully about why you're about to modify your life with. If that item, service or experience is worth it. Then ask yourself:

- Will it feel like a good investment in 90 days, 6 months, or even a year?
- Will it help you create a healthier you?
- Will it help create a happier you?
- Will this change bring you immense joy and memories that will last forever?
- Will you grow as a result?

Investing in your health will have a high return, personally and professionally. Don't go foolishly looking for cheap thrills and expect to be in better state of health this time next year. Believe that you're worthy of investing in yourself and believe you'll have a return.

Notes:

Things We Should Know

I've struggled with body imagine my entire life. I was the skinny girl who you seen eating all the time but I could never gain any weight. I had a very high metabolism. After high school started. I was often teased and harassed, and started to become quite self-conscious about being too skinny. The girls would whisper, giggle and call me names.

Of course, we all have that picture perfect imagine that we want to see when we look in the mirror. For some strange reason we think that our lives would be so much easier, if we could just be "that" size. As women, we seem to allow ourselves to be critiqued by the world's view of our self-image and this can affect our self-esteem.

Love the Skin Your In

You're the only person in this world that is you. You are unique individuals and that is fantastic. Embrace who you are. You are beautiful. You are worthy. You are enough. Accept yourself and love all your flaws.

Find Your Tribe

You are not everyone's cup of tea. We need to feel connected, supported and loved. Finding your tribe of friends will allow you to feel accepted, appreciated and understood. Your tribe will also give you the confidence to stop pretending and be yourself. Keep your standards high, feel good in your own skin and be happy. Soon, you will find yourself surrounded by loving people who will encourage and empower you.

Healthy Habits

Good nutrition is an important part of leading a healthy lifestyle. You can do anything that you set your mind to do. Your new healthy habit can be anything from meditation, eating better or trying out a new exercise. Any decision to improve your overall health will benefit you in the long run. Choose a healthy habit that is easy to start. Remember that your life goals isn't your healthy habit change but it will get you started in the right direction. Don't forget this is all a process. Each day you will become better, stronger and more successful.

Embrace Life

We live in a fast paced superficial world. Where ever you go, there you are. You can't always control the world around you. Take time to breathe everything in, think about what is going on and let circumstances unfold as they may. Why not allow the universe catch you.

Gather Together

I enjoy hanging out with my friends and family over a nice meal. Social connections help us maintain a sense of belonging. Attending a dinner party is heartwarming and it brings people closer. "People with social support have fewer cardiovascular problems and immune problems, and lower levels of cortisol — a stress hormone," says Tasha R. Howe, PhD, associate professor of psychology at Humboldt State University.

Think of Others

Volunteering makes a difference in the lives of other people. Studies have shown that people who volunteer and donate their time feel more socially connected. Many people find volunteer work to be helpful with respect to stress reduction, boost your self-confidence and give you a over satisfaction of happiness. A 2012 study in the journal Health Psychology found that participants who volunteered with some regularity lived longer.

Gratitude

Gratitude means you're thankful for what you have. You count your blessings by noticing the simple pleasures in life. You also acknowledge everything that you receive. You have learned to live your life as if everything was a miracle, and you are aware of everything that have been given to you. Being thankful changes your mindset from what your life lacks to the abundance that you currently have. One way you can start to practice gratitude daily is by keeping a journal of everything in your life that you are thankful to have. Don't wait for something good to happen to practice gratitude. Start seeing the good in every situation. This will help you improve you self-image. It's not what others think about you, it's what you think about yourself that truly matters.

Write down goals

Having hypothyroidism I tend to forget things a lot. I can walk into a room and totally blank out why I went in there in the 1st place. I always make myself a "honey-do" list and check things off as I go throughout my day. A "honey-do" list isn't just for remember things that need to be done. A self-made "honey-do" list can be something you use to write down your goals. Start small by writing down the things you want to eliminate, reduce or cut back on in your life. I know, it's would be silly to think you can accomplish that task in one day but every little bit helps. The more you do the closer you are to obtaining your goal. The more you do, the more often you do them, the healthier and younger you will start to feel.

Plant a garden

Planting a garden is more than just digging in the dirt. It allows you to be one with earth and you are working with living things that you created. Working with our hands it's very beneficial and it allows our mind to destress. We can become one with natural and the world around us.

Speak powerful words to yourself

Be strong, stay positive

Your doctor knows that your hypothyroidism can be an autoimmune disease and the main reason why they don't tell their patients is simple: it has no difference on their treatment plan.

Just because you doctors prescribe it doesn't mean you should take it. You need to research the medications and weigh out your options. Most conventional medicine doesn't effectively treat autoimmune disease. Doctors will use steroids and other medications to suppress the immune system in certain conditions with more potentially damaging effects, such as multiple sclerosis, rheumatoid arthritis and Crohn's disease.

Why wait until the immune system has destroyed the immune system and has destroyed enough thyroid tissue to classify you as hypothyroid? In return give you thyroid hormone replacement pills?

Why not go ahead and start addressing the underlying cause? The immune system attacking the thyroid gland.

Hypothyroidism patients need to understand that they don't have a problem with their thyroid at 1st. They have a problem with their immune system attacking the thyroid. When you immune system is not working properly your thyroid will be affected.

I be able to get off my medication?

Levothyroxine, a synthetic form of thyroid hormone, is the 4th highest selling drug in the U.S. 13 of the top 50 selling drugs are either directly or indirectly related to hypothyroidism. The number of people suffering from thyroid disorders continues to rise each year.

Thyroid medication is only one piece of the puzzle.

Generally, I would be the first person to tell you don't trust pharmaceutical companies. Do your research before you take any medication and out weight the benefits but without sounding like I am contradicting myself. I believe in pharmaceuticals if:

1. They work.

2. They do more good than harm, and;

3. There are no non-drug alternatives with the same effect.

Being on medication isn't a bad thing and I am not saying that everyone with hypothyroid symptoms should be on medication. I want you to understand that when you have elevated TSH this indicates that the body is not producing enough thyroid hormone to meet your metabolic need. Thyroid hormone is very important to the proper function of the body that the sometimes the benefits of replacing it far outweigh any potential side effects of the medication. You can also check with your doctor to see if they offer a natural thyroid medication. One of the biggest problems with thyroid replacement medications are the sensitivities to the fillers used in the medications. Many popular thyroid medications contain common allergens such as cornstarch, dextrose, lactose and even gluten.

This explains why some of us react great to certain thyroid medications and others experience bad side effects.

Richard Shames and Karilee Halo Shames wrote:

Some people do not want to take the time to start with a mild dose, adjusting to their medication gradually. However, we have found that the slow, step-by-step method of reaching your optimal dose is more easily tolerated by the body than the "sock it to me" approach so characteristic of our fast-paced culture.

Slow and steady wins the race. Starting out at a smaller dose and gradually working your way up to the dosage your body needs over a period of time and having regular blood work done sounds like an easier hit on your body.

Meanwhile, during the process of trying to figure out what medication and your right dosage. You can go ahead and start working on finding out what the root cause of your hypothyroidism.

"So let's get back to the work of figuring out how to address the problem naturally."

1. Start eating a hypothyroidism Diet

2. Eat more Iodine rich foods

3. Stay away from Fluoride

4. Dry brush before you shower

Your skin releases toxin through your pores when you sweet but dead skin can clog the pores. You want to brush towards the center of your body in a circular- gentle yet firm round motion.

5. Avoid plastic bottles

Plastic water bottles contain phthalates from the plastic when plastic gets warm these harmful chemicals leach into the water. Phthalates acts like estrogen and throws your hormones out of balance.

6. Replace mercury fillings

7. Avoid Aluminum

8. Exercise Easy

9. Check your stress levels

10. Try to eat organic fruits and vegetables

11. Avoid chemicals

You can start making your own household cleaners. In my book*:* ***Awareness has Magic.*** I have many recipes listed. There are other ways to get rid of weeds and bugs in your home too. Google is a fantastic thing. Google your question and you will find the answer.

Notes:

Did you know that products we use every day may contain toxic chemicals and has been linked to women's health issues? They are hidden endocrine disruptors and are very tricky chemicals that play havoc on our bodies. "We are all routinely exposed to endocrine disruptors, and this has the potential to significantly harm the health of our youth," said Renee Sharp, EWG's director of research. "It's important to do what we can to avoid them, but at the same time we can't shop our way out of the problem. We need to have a real chemical policy reform."

These chemicals will increase production of certain hormones; decreasing production of others; imitating hormones; turning one hormone into another; interfering with hormone signaling; telling cells to die prematurely; competing with essential nutrients; binding to essential hormones; accumulating in organs that produce hormones. You can start avoiding these chemicals by making your own all natural cleaning supplies and being aware of the chemicals that you may purchase for your home, body and yard.

Homemade Deodorant

1/2 cup baking soda

1/2 cup arrowroot powder or 1/2 cup of cornstarch

5 tablespoon unrefined virgin coconut oil

10 drops of grapefruit essential oil or lavender essential oil

(You can pick your favorite scent. I like lavender or grapefruit.)

Mix baking soda and arrowroot together. Melt your coconut oil in the microwave in a microwave-safe bowl. Mix all ingredients (the baking soda and arrowroot powder) with the oil. Pour into clean small Mason jar. Add your essential oil to the Mason jar; close with the lid. Give it a good shake to combine the essential oil with the other mixture. By doing it this way, you can still use that bowl to eat with. Once you mix that essential oil in the bowl, it can only be used for the purpose of making your deodorant. Everything you've used is edible except the essential oils.

There is no one size fits all with Hypothyroidism

I started to research to begin to try to understand that there's really not a one size fits all for us with hypothyroidism but there are certain ways we can eat, things that we need to start incorporating and things we need to start avoiding that will certainly help begin the healing process. Diet alone wasn't enough to help my body start fighting this battle that is raging in your body. I needed to start addressing other areas in your life that can cause inflammation like Dietary Allergies, Addressing gut health and avoiding Chemical toxins and endocrine disruptors. In this book, I have gone in to detail many times over to explain and help guide you on your journey. I am sharing things that I've learned along the way to help you have a smoother transaction that I did. I hope you are taking notes, highlighting and writing along the side of the book. Not everything in this book will affect you directly but it might others. Food is very important part of the healing process. Food not just calories it is information. It talks to your DNA and tells it what to do. My most powerful tool to change my health was my fork. I needed to stop going long periods of time without food. My body always needed energy. If my blood sugar starts to drop this creates a stress reaction and now your adrenal glands will do what it needs to do to maintain my body's function by releasing more cortisol or adrenaline. Eating often would help put your body back in its normal cycle. You need to eat foods that nourish your body and not hinder it.

I really had no idea how powerful food really was until after I was diagnosed with Hypothyroidism. Many people with hypothyroidism are deficient in Magnesium, B-12, Zinc, Iodine, B2, Vitamin C, Selenium, Vitamin D and Vitamin A.

The Standard American diet in a nutshell is loaded with unhealthy saturated and Trans fats. Our meals are unbalanced, over-sized and loaded with sugar, salt, artificial ingredients and preservatives. We have an abundance of food at our finger tips but yet we are extremely malnourished and mineral deficient. We are literally starving our bodies to death! People are not obtaining the basic nutrients their bodies needs in order to fuel what is needed to perform its proper functions. We are literally running on empty! There is about 20 million estimated Americans with some type of hypothyroid disorder.

Although my thyroid is small, it produces a hormone that influences every cell, tissue and organ in the body. My thyroid determines the rate in which my body produces the energy from nutrients and oxygen. So I need to start eating foods that fed my thyroid. I needed to start nourishing my body back to health with foods that jump kicked my metabolism too. After being diagnosed my priorities were made clearer. I had to start listening to my body, stop taking my health for granted and continuing to research to figure out what I needed to do to "fix me". I started making my own cleaning products, lotions and deodorant's. Our skin is the largest organ in our body and it absorbs everything we put on it.

Are you gluten intolerant?

15% of the population is gluten intolerant. 99% of people who either have a gluten intolerance or celiac disease are never diagnosed. More than 55 disease have been linked to the protein found in wheat, rye and barley. Here are a few symptoms that may indicate you have gluten intolerance.

Digestive issues such as gas, bloating, diarrhea and constipation. Keratosis Pilarsis also knows as chicken skin on the back of your arms. Fatigue, brain fog or feeling tired after eating a meal that contains gluten. Migraine headaches. Diagnoses with chronic fatigue or fibromyalgia. Inflammation, swelling or pain in your joints, hips, knees and fingers. Mood issues such as anxiety, ADD, depression and mood swings. Hormone imbalances such as PMS, PCOS or unexplained infertility. Diagnoses of autoimmune disease such as Hashimoto Thyroiditis, rheumatoid arthritis, ulcerative colitis, lupus, psoriasis and scleroderma.

Gluten is that protein that is found in wheat and other grains and it will pass through the lining of your gut and into your blood stream, your immune system will tag the foreign invader (gluten) with antibodies for destruction. When you are gluten intolerant this will cause a problem where your immune system can mistake the thyroid for gluten, causing it to come under attack.

Remember gluten is an inflammatory for the gut and should be removed from the diet of anyone with autoimmune disorders.

There's Magic in the Mud

I haven't used store bought toothpaste in years. I didn't give up brushing my teeth although sometimes I would like to create my very own six foot "personal space bubble." My teeth are beautifully white and my breath is always fresh. After being diagnosed with hypothyroidism, I started researching and was amazed at the things we willingly without even thinking put in or on our bodies that are very harmful to us. I started to take a closer look at all the labels of EVERYTHING and decided that I needed to divorce my store bought toothpaste.

Did you know that your teeth are living and spongy? The foods we eat, the commercial toothpastes, medications and chemicals from drinks all can suck out the minerals from the teeth causing weakened enamel and leaving us more susceptible to decay and breakdown. I was on a new mission to keep my teeth healthy by using the absolute necessary and needed trace minerals to maintain the upmost dental health plus find a solution that wasn't abrasive, while gently polishing them, and detoxifies while it refreshes. Is there such a thing? I did know that my long history with Mr. Store bought toothpaste were over.

Sorry, Mr. Toothpaste. I thought we were great together but actually you're sucking the life out of me. So, it's not me. It's you, and here's why:

Did you know that fluoride was Once Prescribed as an Anti-Thyroid Drug? Up through the 1950s, doctors in Europe and South America prescribed fluoride to reduce thyroid function in patients with over-active thyroids (hyperthyroidism). (Merck Index 1968).   If you haven't already, you should invest in a water filtration system to rid your tap water of fluoride. Do we really know how safe tap water is? Look at the recent events in Flint Michigan! Can you really trust the water companies? Although fluoride concentrations in tap water are relatively low and are considered "safe" for human consumption, it is not. Fluoride has long-term neurological and hormonal affects. Fluoride is not an essential nutrient. It is also that chemical that is commonly found in most toothpaste brands. There is clear evidence that, when ingested at high doses, fluoride causes neurotoxicity. Fluoride also is understood to interfere with the absorption of iodine, possibly leading to an iodine deficiency and ultimately hypothyroidism. To benefit your health, use fluoride free tooth or make your own tooth paste. Get a good water filtration system and purchase a filter for your shower head. We use a British Berkefeld.

Store bought toothpaste also have other ingredients in it like:

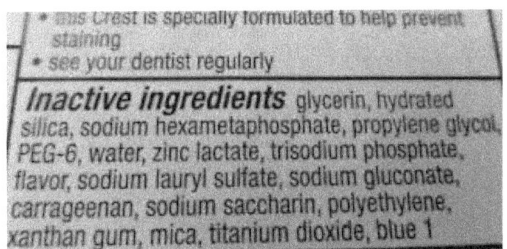

Glycerin is used in almost all toothpastes because it helps create a pasty texture and prevents it from drying out. Although it's non-toxic it coats the teeth just enough to that prevents normal tooth remineralization. Remineralization is a whole-body process and in order for it to happen, the body must have adequate levels of certain nutrients, especially fat soluble vitamins and certain minerals. If you want to stop and reverse Tooth Decay you must add minerals in your diet, add plenty of fat soluble vitamins (A, D, E and K), and your body must be able to absorb vital nutrients. You certainly can't do this by having a coat on your teeth that will prevent absorption.

Sodium Lauryl Sulfate (SLS) is a foaming agent and detergent that is commonly used in toothpaste, shampoo, and other products such as degreaser for car engines. SLS is an estrogen mimicker. It also increases gum inflammation and mouth ulcers. According to a study conducted the Department of Oral Surgery & Oral Medicine in Oslo, Norway, individuals who used a toothpaste containing SLS suffered from more ulcers (canker sores) than those who used an SLS-free toothpaste.

Sweeteners: Sorbitol, sodium saccharin and other artificial sweeteners are often used in toothpaste to improve taste, even though there is no evidence that these sweeteners are beneficial (or even safe) for use in the mouth. Xylitol has shown some positive benefits for oral health in some studies, but it remains a controversial ingredient in toothpaste.

Triclosan: A chemical used in antibacterial soaps and products. Triclosan was recently found to affect proper heart function in a study at University of California Davis and the FDA is currently re-evaluating it for safety in human use.

Let's not forget to mention that many toothpastes also contain artificial colors/dyes or synthetic flavors. I must admit there are several good natural toothpastes out there and I have tried some of them not all but with my tight budget I will make them for pennies on the dollar. My favorite way to brush my teeth is by using tooth powder. Yes, you read this right. Tooth Powder. Here is my recipe that I use. Feel free to adjust the ingredient's based on your own needs. If you have sensitive teeth you might want to skip the baking soda and salt until you can get used to it.

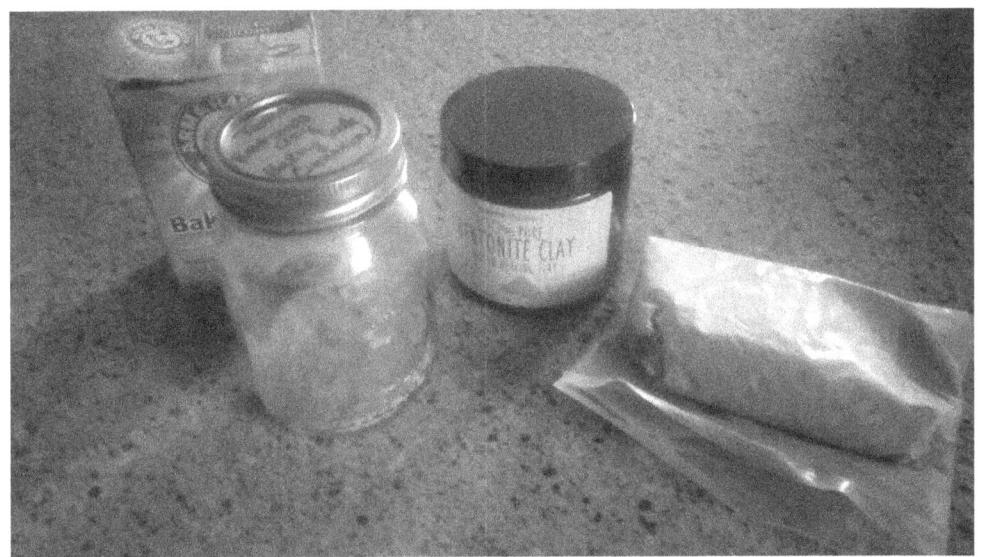

Homemade Tooth Powder Recipe

Ingredients

- 4 tablespoons Bentonite Clay
- 2 teaspoons baking soda
- 1 ½ teaspoons finely ground unrefined sea salt
- ½ teaspoons clove powder
- 1 teaspoon ground Ceylon cinnamon

- 5-10 drops of peppermint essential oil
- ¾ teaspoons activated charcoal – optional

Directions:

Using a stainless steel or plastic spoon, mix all ingredients in a clean glass jar. To use, add a little to a wet toothbrush and brush as normal.

Bentonite Clay

Bentonite clay is a gentle cleanser that is rich in minerals which support tooth remineralization. Its detoxifying properties help freshen breath and fight gum disease, while it's adsorptive properties help remove stains from teeth.

Baking Soda

Baking soda is a mild abrasive tooth polish that helps mechanically remove stains while other ingredients such as clay and activated charcoal draw them out. It also helps freshen breath.

Sea Salt

Unrefined sea salts such as this one contain 60+ trace minerals that aid in tooth remineralization. Salt is also highly antiseptic, which helps keep bacteria in check.

Herb & Spices

Spices and herbs such as clove powder, ground cinnamon, and ground mint add flavoring, but they also have astringent properties that support gum health.

Activated Charcoal

Activated carbon – is made by processing charcoal with oxygen and either calcium chloride or zinc chloride. It was used medicinally by both Hippocrates and the ancient Egyptians, and it is still the poison remedy of choice in modern day emergency rooms. Why? Because it's highly adsorptive, which in plain English means it attracts substances to its surface like a magnet. Like absorptive substances which work like a sponge, adsorptive materials bind with certain compounds and prevent our bodies from using them.

If you're not so hip on using powdered tooth then here are some more all natural recipes.

Natural Peppermint Toothpaste

1/2 cup coconut oil

3 Tablespoons of baking soda

15 drops of peppermint food grade essential oil

Melt to soften the coconut oil. Mix in other ingredients and stir well. Place your mixture into small glass jar. Allow it to cool completely. When ready to use just dip toothbrush in and scrape small amount onto bristles.

Homemade Coconut Oil Toothpaste Recipe

6 tbsp. coconut oil

6 tbsp. baking soda

15-20 drops of a food grade essential oil (peppermint essential oil)

Melt to soften the coconut oil. Mix in other ingredients and stir well. Place your mixture into small glass jar. Allow it to cool completely. When ready to use just dip toothbrush in and scrape small amount onto bristles.

Chapter 4

Thyroid Hormones:

The Thyroid hormones control the functions of every single cell in your body. These hormones play a crucial role in supporting the functions of the brain, heart, lungs, the gut, bones, joints muscles and skin.

You shouldn't be a bit surprised when an under-functioning thyroid gland may help offer with a variation of symptoms and physical changes that manifest due to the breakdown of any of these body parts.

People are affected with fatigue, weight gain, muscle and joint pains, dry skin, hair loss, digestive complaints, depressive moods, brain fog and poor concentration, breathing difficulties, headaches, sleep disturbances, dry eyes and hearing loss may all be related to an under-functioning thyroid gland.

Although you lab results may be normal you still have all these symptoms.

Now once you do start taking medication you might have a whole new list of issues to add like weight gain, chronic fatigue, mood swings, mental lethargy, lethargy, muscles pains, the continuation of brain fog and dry skin.

Getting on the Right Medication

How do you know if you are on the right type of thyroid medication?

Let's discuss a few important things without it sounding like a foreign unknown language:

There are two forms of thyroid hormone floating around in your body.

1. T4 or Thyroxine - This is the carrier form of thyroid hormone. T4 is a hormone has a role in many of the body functions, including growth and metabolism. There are two kinds of T4 tests: a total T4 test and a free T4 test. A number of drugs can interfere with your T4 levels, so tell your doctor what medications you're taking before a T4 test. T4. Some of your T4 is called free T4. Free T4 doesn't bond well to protein in your blood. Most of the T4 in your body does bond with protein.

2. T3 or Triiodothyronine - This is the active form of thyroid hormone and the majority in your body comes from T4 conversion to T3. T4 can turn into either the active T3 or the inactive reverse T3.

Many doctors give out T4 only medication and hope that your body will have no problem converting the T4 into the active thyroid hormone T3. Sometimes there isn't a problem and T4 medication works perfectly fine.

Contrary to the old ways on the process of shifting the T4 into T3 is constrained by a number of things that affect thyroid overall function which are: Stress, Insulin resistance, Leptin resistance, Prescription medications and Chemical toxins.

Some patients seem to do better on some form of T3 (triiodothyronine) added to their current thyroid medication.

Thyroid medication options:

1. T4 only medications

Synthroid (Levothyroxine), Levoxyl, Tirosint

Synthroid T4 only medication

Levoxyl t4 only medication

Tirosint t4 medication

2. T3 only medications

Cytomel (liothyronine) or Sustained Release T3 (from compounding pharmacy)

liothyronine t3 only medication

3. Combination of T3 and T4 medications

Natural Dessicated Thyroid - Armour Thyroid, Westhroid, Naturethroid, etc.

Combinations of T4 and T3: Cytomel + Synthroid or Combos from compounding pharmacies.

Armour Thyroid compounded T4 and T3

Westhroid combo of T4 and T3 medication

Naturethroid combo t4 and t3 medication

If you are on a T4 only medication (like Synthroid or levothyroxine) and you are still symptomatic, it might benefit you if you add some form of T3. Then again, your medication could be exactly what you need but you're not addressing other issues like for instance your gut health, environmental toxins, eating right, your stress, your sleep or even other medications that you are taking. This isn't a one size fits all fix. You must start working on other area's in your life too. If you want to get better.

Some people do decide to take Natural Dessicated Thyroid (NDT), and other people do require higher amounts of T3 only medication and benefit from taking Cytomel alone or a combination of Cytomel and Synthroid together.

Remember we are all individual's. The type of thyroid medication and the dose you need will depend solely on your own body. Don't assume that if a certain medication worked for Sally it will work for you.

Trial and error, along with blood work, how you feel and paying attention to your symptoms are the best way to find your type of medication and dosage.

Thyroid Resistance and Reverse T3

Thyroid resistance is a recently new term that means that your cells are resistant to thyroid hormone. Sounds crazy, huh?

Hopefully, I won't make you fall asleep or completely confuse you with this. So here goes.

Your body adapts T4 to the inactive hormone reverse T3. If you have too much reverse T3 in your blood, it will sit on top of the T3 receptor and blocks T3 from entering the cells. Sounds strange doesn't it? Reverse T3 is the "bully" form of the T3 hormone. Blood work will be able to determine if you have higher levels of reverse T3. In which all you have to do to fix this is add more T3 hormone and cut back on your T4 medications.

Your Thyroid Medications isn't working

I need for you to understand that you have to start addressing the root of your hypothyroidism. Just taking thyroid medication is a band-aide solution to putting your hypothyroidism in remission. After you've been diagnosed with Hypothyroidism it means that your thyroid isn't producing the needed thyroid hormone for your body to properly function.

It is important to understand if you have inflammation in your body it will suppress your thyroid hormones and also decreases the responsiveness of thyroid receptors. Look at it this way. You can be dedicated in never missing a dose of thyroid medication and you can also be on the correct dosage as well but if your thyroid cell receptors are blocking the medication to enter due to inflammation that is suppressing your thyroid it's like moving 2 steps forward and 1 step back.

Another thing, if you have inflammation it decreases the conversion of T4 (inactive thyroid hormone) to T3 (active form of thyroid hormone). So if you're only taking the synthetic hormone medicines (Synthroid, Unithroid, Levoxyl, etc.) which are only T4, and you have inflammation, it won't work at all because it can't be converted to the active form. To start to restore balance in your body, you must 1st start addressing your hypothyroidism by fixing your immune system and the inflammation that could be raging in your body. Let's not forget that sugar and processed foods can lead to increased inflammation in the body. You must start using more natural remedies while fighting hypothyroidism. The SAD (standard American Diet) is such a poor diet that stresses our bodies more and keeps us lacking the vital nutrients that we need.

I've learned to take my medication as soon as I get up along with a warm lemon water with my thyroid medication.

Lemons are loaded with healthy benefits, and particularly, they're a great vitamin C food source. One cup of fresh lemon juice provides 187 percent of your daily recommended serving of vitamin C — take that, oranges! Lemon juice also offers up a healthy serving of potassium, magnesium and copper.

It Aids in digestion and detoxification. It tricks the liver into producing bile, which helps keep food moving through your body and gastrointestinal tract smoothly. Lemon water also helps relieve indigestion or ease an upset stomach.

I've also learned to wait 1 hour before I eat and wait 4 hours before you take any other vitamin supplements because it can interfere with the absorption of your medication. I've also found out that If I wanted to drink coffee I must wait 1 hour after I've taken my medication because it can also interfere with the absorption of your thyroid medication and to never ever to forget to eat breakfast! I need fuel but I have to wait 1 hour after I've taken my thyroid pill.

Did you know that some medicines can interfere with thyroid hormone production and lead to hypothyroidism, including

- *amiodarone, a heart medicine*
- *interferon alpha, a cancer medicine*
- *lithium, a bipolar disorder medicine*
- *interleukin-2, a kidney cancer medicine*

What Tests Should I Request?

Many cases of thyroid problems can be missed because some won't doctors perform a complete comprehensive thyroid test panel. There are some doctors who will only test your TSH.   Here is a list of tests that you can take to your doctor and request. They will not only test for Hashimoto's and hypothyroidism but other things that might be affecting your health. Be sure to request a copy of your thyroid labs so that you can see them yourself and ensure that they are understood accurately.

1. TSH (Thyroid Stimulating Hormone)

TSH - This is a pituitary hormone that responds to low/high amounts of thyroid hormone that is moving around in your blood stream. In some cases of Hashimoto's and primary hypothyroidism, this lab test will be elevated. In the case of Graves' disease the TSH will be low. People with Hashimoto's and central hypothyroidism may have a normal reading on this test.

2. Thyroid peroxidase antibodies (TPO Antibodies) & Thyroglobulin Antibodies (TG Antibodies)
3. Thyroid peroxidase antibodies (TPO Antibodies) and Thyroglobulin Antibodies (TG Antibodies) - People with Hashimoto's will have an elevation of one or both of these antibodies.
4. Free T3 & Free T4

Free T3 & Free T4 - These tests measure the levels of active thyroid hormone moving around in the body.

5. Reverse T3
6. Basic Metabolic Panel
7. Ferritin level (iron)

You also want to check to see if you have any nutrient deficiencies. The most common nutrient deficiencies are Protein, Magnesium, B-12, Zinc, Iodine, B2, Vitamin C, Selenium, Vitamin D, Vitamin A and iron. So, don't allow your doctor to perform a standard TSH test. Those in itself are simply unreliable. You want to have vitamin panels, hormone panels, candida test, Lyme tests, and adrenal tests too. The best way to prevent a deficiency is to eat a balanced, real food-based diet that includes nutrient-dense foods (both plants and animals).

Chapter 5
Adopting a Hypothyroidism Diet

Many people underestimate the importance in which their diet can have a direct effect on their thyroid levels. Eating certain foods can affect how well your body is able to absorb vital nutrients. A hypothyroidism diet is unlikely to "cure" hypothyroidism but it will certainly help to will reduce your symptoms. Eating certain foods and/or certain drinks (e.g. coffee) along with your medication can interfere with how your body reacts to the absorption and subsequently can change your thyroid levels. Most people with hypothyroidism are nutrient deficient, chemically toxic, and have a cortisol overload. Eating more nutrient-dense foods, reducing sugar intake, avoiding soy, making your own cleaning chemicals and avoiding preservatives may prove beneficial for overall health. Feeding your body with nutrient dense foods provides significant benefit in thyroid function and your hormonal biomarkers. Hormones are these little chemical messengers that are produced in one part of the body and released into the blood to trigger or regulate particular functions in other parts of your body. Your endocrine system is the supervisor. It's in charge of these network of glands throughout the body that regulate certain body functions, including body temperature, metabolism, growth, and sexual development. Understand that there are things that individually help to halter your thyroid ability to absorb your medication and you need specific foods to improve thyroid function. Our thyroid plays a most important role in metabolism. Along with your insulin and cortisol levels, thyroid hormones are an accelerating force behind metabolic rate and weight management. Many health problems start to appear if our thyroid stops working properly. Diet alone won't cure your hypothyroidism. Improving your dietary consumption by eating food that feed and heal your thyroid may also enhance T4 and T3 levels.

Why should I care about eating to cater to my thyroid?
Why all have to die someday.

Sometimes I want to shake people and say "Wake up!" You have to power to make a difference. You've always had the power. No one can force you to eat processed foods. Eating healthy isn't easy. Adjusting your life and catering to your specific health needs will benefit you in the long run. This is one of the smartest decisions that you can make. Not only will you start to look and feel better but think of the medical costs that you could be saving your future self. Not having the right nourishment makes your body sluggish, exhausted, and week. No one but you can do this. You have to be your own health advocate. Do you ever wonder what are the reasons why people are getting sick are? What is the real reason? Could it be pollution? Could it be radiation from cellular devices? Could it be global warming? Could it be lack of nutrients in our farming soil or pesticides in our food? Could it be the sneaky hidden sugars in our foods along with the saturated fat, extra sodium and tons of empty calories we consume mindlessly? No wonder our bodies are sick. The nutrients in food allow the cells in our bodies to perform their necessary functions. In other words, nutrients give our bodies instructions about how to function.

Here is a list of the top 4 causes of death in the United States. This is a statistic report from 2007 taken from the National Vital Statistics Report. None of these things may affect you directly but I am sure you know someone who it has. These numbers should scare you. You could be next.

There were total of 2,423,712 reported deaths in the United States in 2007.

1. Diseases of heart (heart disease)- 616,067 – 25.4 % of total deaths in 2007

2. Malignant neoplasms (cancer) – 562,875 – 23.2 % of total deaths in 2007

3. Cerebrovascular diseases (stroke) – 135,952

4. Chronic lower respiratory diseases – 127,924

Can I scream this louder!?

EVERY CELL IN YOUR BODY CAN BE IMPACTED BY THYROID MALFUNCTION

The Recipes

All of the recipes in every one of my books are catered towards healing your thyroid. Cruciferous vegetables are excellent for your health it has been proven to interfere with thyroid function when eaten raw. Please limit your cooked cruciferous vegetable intake to 2x a week until you get your thyroid working at the optimum level again. Cruciferous vegetables are rich sources of sulfur-containing compounds known as glucosinolates. Some glucosinolates found in raw cruciferous vegetables produces a compound known as goitrin, which has been found to interfere with thyroid hormone production. Very high intakes of raw cruciferous vegetables, such as raw cabbage and raw turnips, have been found to cause hypothyroidism. The reason for this book is give you the tools you need so you're not in the kitchen cooking 3 different meals. All the recipes are nutrient packed to supply your thyroid with the help is needs to support your thyroid plus everyone will enjoy them. Your family will think you're a master in the kitchen!

People with hypothyroidism may feel that they have a limited selection of foods but you don't! Remember food is information. It's more than just calories. The type of food you eat will determine if you're to be healthy or sick. You must tailor your nutritional needs to your body. Being on a very restrictive diet when you don't to be can put you at risk for adrenal fatigue and nutrient deficiencies.

A diet for hypothyroidism should include whole foods rich in iodine:

whole baked organic potatoes with skin, cod, dried seaweed, shrimp, Himalayan crystal salt, baked turkey breast, dried prunes, navy beans, tuna, boiled eggs, lobster, cranberries, and green beans. Niacin-rich foods (required for normal manufacture of thyroid hormone) are tuna, chicken, prunes, bananas, turkey, salmon, sardines, and brown rice.

Riboflavin-rich foods:

Raw almonds, eggs, mushrooms, sesame seeds, salmon, and tuna.

Zinc: (as well as vitamins B6, C, and E, iodine) is a major component of thyroid hormone balance and is antimicrobial. Zinc-rich foods (boost thyroid function) are white cooked button mushrooms, chickpeas, kidney beans, dark chocolate (70 percent or higher), pumpkin, squash seeds, and almonds.

Selenium-rich foods: (helps to convert T-4 to T-3) are Brazil nuts and tuna.

High-polyphenols foods: (acts as an anti-fungal) are cocoa powder, dark chocolate, coffee, tea, flaxseed meal, red raspberries, blueberries, black currants.

Vitamin B6–rich foods: (required for normal manufacture of thyroid hormone) are raw unsalted sunflower seeds, quinoa, raw pumpkin seeds, sesame seeds, flaxseeds, pistachio nuts, cashews, tuna, halibut, salmon, dried prunes, bananas, avocados, dried apricots, and raisins.

Vitamin C–rich foods: (boost thyroid gland function) are bell peppers, dark leafy greens, kiwis, broccoli, berries, citrus fruits, tomatoes, peas, and papayas.

Riboflavin-rich foods: (or vitamin b2—essential for normal manufacture of thyroid hormone) are frozen peas, beets, crimini mushrooms, eggs, asparagus, almonds, and turkey.

Vitamin E–rich foods: (work with zinc and vitamin A to produce thyroid hormone) are raw almonds, shrimp, avocados, quinoa, salmon, extra-virgin olive oil, and cooked butternut squash.

See you are NOT limited to what you can eat with hypothyroidism. You have many options to what you can eat and why you need to be eating this. Here are more foods and YES you may read repeats from the paragraph above but I want you to see what an abundance of foods that you can eat. The only limit you have in the kitchen is your imagination. My recipes are a starting point. You can start to creating your favorite recipes and healing your thyroid as you eat! Your diet is part of the solution.

Fatty fish like wild salmon, trout, halibut, cod, albacore tuna, flounder, cod or sardines (omega-3s and selenium) only a few times per week....

No farmed fish, period!

No gluten.

Split peas, lentils, black beans, kidney beans, pinto beans, artichokes, raspberries, blackberries, chia seeds, red apples with skin, prunes, green peas, raw almonds, garbanzo beans, winter squash, spaghetti squash, summer squash, butternut squash, zucchini, popcorn (no microwave-ready, bagged popcorn), cherries, citrus fruits, kiwi, cantaloupe, papaya, mango, plums and red grapes, tomatoes, carrots, gluten-free, steel-cut oats or gluten-free rolled oats, watermelon, green tea, organic apple cider vinegar, lemon, garlic, leeks, parsley, celery, ginger root, tomatoes, cucumbers, carrots, asparagus, organic whole baked potatoes with skin, shrimp, Himalayan crystal salt, Celtic sea salt, baked turkey breast, dried prunes, navy beans, gluten free steel cut or rolled oats, cranberries and green beans, organic no hormone chicken, brown rice, raw almonds, eggs, sesame seeds,, chickpeas, kidney beans, dark chocolate 70 percent or higher, walnuts, cocoa powder, hempseeds, red raspberries, blueberries, black currants, brazil nuts, raw unsalted sunflower seeds, quinoa, raw pumpkin seeds, sesame seeds, flaxseeds, pistachio nuts, cashews, dried prunes, bananas, avocados, dried apricots, and raisins, red, green and orange bell peppers, romaine lettuce, kiwis, papayas, beets, all mushrooms, quinoa, extra-virgin olive oil and cooked butter nut squash. sea vegetables, dried seaweed, kelp, dulse, nori, arame, wakame, kombu, tomato paste, brewer's yeast, brown rice, algae, healing spices (Ceylon cinnamon, turmeric, gloves, cayenne pepper, garlic, oregano, sage, ginger .

Let's talk about legumes.

Green beans, Navy beans, Lentils, chickpeas and kidney beans are in the legume family and are very good for your thyroid unless you have a food allergy. These beans are a rich in Iodine and an excellent source of fiber. Total dietary fiber intake should be 25 to 30 grams a day from food, not supplements. Are you getting your daily intake? Probably not, so these beans that I have listed are an excellent choice to add to your plate. Soy & peanuts are also legumes and I never-ever suggest those.

Always AVOID SOY

You must be confused about soy as so much has been said about this little bean. Well, if you have a thyroid condition, it's likely that your hormonal health overall has been compromised. It's best to avoid soy as it elevates the estrogen levels.

Food to avoid: tofu, soymilk, soy lecithin (used as fillers in f.eg veggie burgers), and soy oil.

Fermented soy like miso and tempeh are OK though. Always pick non-GMO (non-genetically modified) and MSG-free miso and tempeh)

Soy products have hormone disrupting effects. Soy is also high in isoflavones (or goitrogens), which can damage your thyroid gland. Products containing soy protein appear in nearly every aisle of the supermarket. That's because soy doesn't just mean tofu. Traditional soy foods also include soymilk, soynuts and edamame (green soybeans), just to name a few. Food companies also develop new food products containing soy protein from veggie burgers to fortified pastas and cereals. READ your labels. Don't worry you still can eat fried brown rice but replace it with Coconut amino's instead. Soy is estrogen mimicking, goitrogenic, hexane filled, protease inhibiting, GMO & a environmental destroying food."

Fermented Foods

A healthy gut plays a significant role in hormone regulation. Having a leaky gut or a lack of probiotic foods lining your intestinal wall can help cause a hormonal imbalance. For most of us, taking a quality probiotic supplement doesn't have any side effects other than higher energy and better digestive health. As a society we have drastically cut back on our consumption of vegetables and of beneficial essential fatty acids (flax, pumpkin, black current seed oil, dark green leafy vegetables, hemp, chia seeds, fish) such as those found in certain fish (including salmon, mackerel, and herring) and flaxseed. We are consume little fiber to no fiber and eat an excess of sugar, salt, and processed foods. Stress, changes in the diet, contaminated food, chlorinated water, and numerous other factors can also alter the bacterial flora in the intestinal tract. When you treat the whole person instead of just treating a disease or symptom, an imbalance in the intestinal tract stands out like an elephant in the room. So to play it safe, I recommend taking a probiotic supplement every. Along with eating fermented foods.

Probiotics are live bacteria and yeasts that are good for your health, especially your digestive system. Probiotics are often called "good" or "helpful" bacteria because they help keep your gut healthy. Probiotics foods include yogurt, kefir, Kimchi, Sour Pickles (brined in water and sea salt instead of vinegar) Pickle juice is rich in electrolytes, and has been shown to help relieve exercise-induced muscle cramps., Kombucha, kombucha tea ,Fermented meat, fish, and eggs.

Prebiotics foods are brown rice, oatmeal, flax, chia, asparagus, Raw Jerusalem artichokes, leeks, artichokes, garlic, carrots, peas, beans, onions, chicory, jicama, tomatoes, frozen bananas, cherries, apples, pears, oranges, strawberries, cranberries, kiwi, and berries are good sources. Nuts are also a prebiotic source. All these foods that I have listed is hypothyroidism friendly.

The ideal pH for the colon is very slightly acidic, in the 6.7–6.9 range. When there is an imbalance or lack of beneficial bacteria in the colon, the pH is typically more alkaline, around 7.5 or higher. The optimal pH range for gas-producing organisms is slightly alkaline at 7.2–7.3.

When someone starts taking a probiotic or a prebiotic supplement (or eats a prebiotic food), the beneficial microorganisms begin to increase in number. These good bacteria start to ferment more soluble fiber into beneficial products like butyric acid, acetic acid, lactic acid, and propionic acid. These acids provide energy, improve mineral, vitamin, and fat absorption, and help prevent inflammation and cancer. The extra acid also starts to lower the pH in the colon.

Homemade Raw Kombucha Fermented Applesauce

Ingredients

5-6 apples

1/4 cup kombucha - can be plain or flavored.

Instructions

Peel, core, and slice apples. Place in food processor and puree. Add kombucha and puree until you reach desired consistency. Place in sealed mason jar and leave on the counter for 24 hours. Store in fridge. This will stay good for 1 month.

Natural Hormone Balancing

One approach to fixing thyroid issues and hypothyroidism is the use of hormone therapy. You really need to meet with a holistic expert. There are many great holistic and naturopath doctors. Most often, synthetic hormones like Synthroid, Levoxyl, or Levothroid are used, which contain only the T4 hormone and no T3 – two hormones produced by the thyroid gland. Thyroid conditions are serious business. You should always seek a professional who knows how to help you. Our organs and glands like your thyroid, adrenals, pituitary, ovaries, testicles and pancreas regulate most of your hormone production, and if your hormones become even slightly imbalanced it can cause some other serious health issues. Our gut health can also play an important role in hormone regulation. Start loading up on up on rich sources of natural omega-3s like wild fish, flaxseed, chia seeds, walnuts and grass-fed animal products. People don't boost their omega-3 foods intake to balance out the elevated omega-6s they consumed. To many mega-6 foods will cause inflammation and lead to chronic disease. Eating more coconut oil, salmon, grass fed butt like Ghee and avocados will start to provide your body with essential fats that are fundamental building blocks for hormone production. Supplements like digestive enzymes, probiotics, bone broth, kefir, fermented vegetables, and high-fiber foods can start to repair your gut lining, which also can help to balance your hormones. Caffeine will rise your cortisol levels and then it lowers your thyroid hormone levels and basically creates havoc throughout your entire body. Replace your morning coffee with herbal teas. Matcha tea is a great caffeine replacement and is loaded with antioxidants, weight loss benefits, and cancer fighting properties, heart health, brain power, skin health and a good Chlorophyll Source. Last but not least GET OUT IN THE SUN! Free vitamin D, baby. 20 minutes a day is a great way to soak up some that free essential vitamin. On the days where you can't sit out in the sun you can supplement with a good D3 vitamin.

Beauty Tip!

Mediating and looking more Toned

Any time you change your diet from unhealthy to a healthier way of eating you should always exercise to help release toxins that have been sitting in your body from years of improper digestion, preservatives from our foods , poisons in our skin care products, pollutions, house hold chemicals , stress and along with other things. Sweating when you exercise is one way to cleanse your body and help release those toxins that has built up in your body. Yoga is wonderful to help tone, slows your mind process down and relieves stress. A nice steamed sauna is excellent to help pull out those toxins too. My local YMCA has a steam sauna room and I use it frequently. Our body is a wonderful, fantastic thing. It has its own eliminative organs which include the lungs, liver kidneys, colon, and your skin. Sometimes you will notice detoxing changes in the way of acne, rashes, colds and flu. When this happens what do we normally do? Take medications to fix it or put medications on it. Why not fix the root of the issue instead of covering up the issue. Your body is trying to tell you it's overloaded with toxicity. What you do? You can start eating right. Be mindful of what you put in your mouth. Before you take that next bite ask yourself: How is this feeding my body with nutrients? Remember, with every bite of food you consume your either fighting disease or feeding disease. Once you start on this journey. You might feel a bit more bloated, a headache, even a skin rash, aches and pains, soreness and moodiness. Don't be alarmed and this is only temporary. All those years of toxic build up in your body is making its way out of your body! Stay strong you will feel and look incredible and your body will be thanking you. So will those jeans too!

Notes:

Start Supporting your Adrenal Glands

Your adrenals produce over 50 hormones that tell almost every bodily function what they need to be doing. These hormones affect every function, organ and tissue in the body. Eating refined foods and sugars will cause a spike in your blood sugar levels, which in return cause the body to release insulin and as a result the adrenal glands will release more cortisol. When you adrenal glands are compromised this puts your body in a catabolic state. Which means your body is breaking down. Since your thyroid glands controls the metabolic activity of the body, it will attempt to slow down the catabolic state by slowing down your metabolism.

You need to start adding nutrient-dense foods that are easy to digest and have healing qualities such as

- Coconut
- Olives
- Avocado
- Cruciferous vegetables (cauliflower, broccoli, Brussels sprouts, etc.) Cooked.... (Limit 2x week)
- Fatty fish (e.g., wild-caught salmon)
- Chicken and turkey
- Nuts, such as walnuts and almonds

- Seeds, such as pumpkin, chia and flax
- Kelp and seaweed
- Celtic or Himalayan sea salt

Low-glycemic veggies (more than 6 servings per day, remember crueferious veggies no more than 2x week)

Artichokes, Artichoke hearts, Asparagus, Bamboo shoots, Bean sprouts, **Broccoli, Brussels sprouts, Cauliflower**, Celery, Cucumber, Daikon, Eggplant, Leeks, Lentils, Beans (green, kidney, garbanzo), Greens (**collard, kale, mustard, turnip**),Mushrooms, Okra, Onions, Pea pods, Peppers, **Radishes**, Rutabaga, Squash, Sugar snap peas, **Swiss chard**, Tomato, Water chestnuts, **Watercress,** Zucchini, **Cabbage (green, bok choy, Chinese)**Salad greens (chicory, endive, escarole, iceberg lettuce, romaine, **spinach, arugula, radicchio, watercress**)

Low- Glycemic fruits (no more than 1 serving per day)

- Eat real food—not processed foods
- Try to eat as organically as possible.
- If you're unable to eat organically, try to eat as naturally as possible.
- Buy organic free range eggs

Coconut oil

Raw, Virgin Coconut oil has been used as just one hypothyroidism natural treatment. Coconut oil is made up of medium chain fatty acids known as medium chain triglyceride's (MCTs), which help with metabolism and weight loss, coconut oil can also raid basal body temperatures – all good news for people suffering from low thyroid function.

Should I oil pull?

Coconut Oil pulling can really transform your health. Your mouth is the home to millions of bacteria, fungi, viruses and other toxins, the oil acts like a cleanser, pulling out the nasties before they get a chance to spread throughout the body.

 This frees up the immune system, reduces stress, curtails internal inflammation and aids well-being.

An ancient Ayurveda ritual dating back over 3,000 years, oil pulling involves placing a tablespoon of extra virgin organic cold pressed oil (I use coconut oil) into your mouth and then swishing it around for up to 20 minutes, minimum 5 minutes (pulling it between your teeth), before spitting it out. Whatever you do, do not swallow the oil as you will ingest the toxins you are trying to wipe out. Afterwards requires brushing your teeth with an all-natural fluoride-free toothpaste, and rinsing your mouth out. And you're done! It really is that easy.

Because coconut oil has been shown to:

- Balance Hormones
- Kill Candida
- Improve Digestion
- Moisturize Skin
- Reduce Cellulite
- Decrease Wrinkles and Age Spots
- Balance Blood Sugar and Improve Energy

- Improve Alzheimer's
- Increase HDL and Lower LDL Cholesterol

Reading Labels

Start reading product labels. You will be surprised where soy, high fructose corn syrup and additives are hiding.

What do we need to do to start healing our hypothyroidism? Let's go over a few things that I've written that are very important things you should know.

The most common allergies and food intolerances are from gluten and dairy (A1 Casein). These proteins are far from simple and can cause a "Leaky Gut" which in return will cause inflammation in your body. The only safe dairy products to consume are from A2 cows, goat milk, sheep milk or nut milks. Gluten creates a havoc in the gut (where the immune system lives) by creating and weakens your immune system.

Start drinking from glass, stainless steel, or BPA free plastic bottles. Bisphenol A (BPA) is found in plastic bottles and can damage your endocrine system and this will have an effect on your thyroid.

Foods, Supplements, and Medication Interactions

When it comes to thyroid medications, it's important for you to know the medications can interact with common nutritional supplements. Calcium supplements have the potential to interfere with proper absorption of your thyroid medications. Wait 4 hours after your thyroid medication before you take anything with calcium in it.

As I've already mentioned in this book that coffee lowers the absorption of your thyroid medication, therefore you need to wait 1 hour before you enjoy that 1st cup. This also goes hand in hand for a fiber supplement.

If you are taking Chromium picolinate, which is marketed for blood sugar control and weight loss, this also interferes with the absorption of your thyroid medications. You should wait four hours between the medications.

Start adding a sprinkle of dulse flakes to your food. Most people with hypothyroidism has low Iodine levels. Kelp and seaweed products can certainly boost your iodine levels. If you start taking a liquid iodine supplement make sure you're under a doctor's care.

Start adding some Milk Thistle, Turmeric, Chlorella, and Cilantro to your smoothies or plate. These food items with help detox harmful metals from your cells and organs.

Start eating more brazil nuts, salmon, sunflower seeds, grass fed beef, mushrooms and onions this is a natural way to get more selenium in your diet.

Get some sun! Vitamin D is often very low with people who have hypothyroidism. You can also start eating more foods like salmon, oysters and sardines. You can add a D3 fermented fish or cod liver supplement. Try to avoid synthetic vitamin D-fortified foods or drinks. **Go for the real stuff.**

Start eating lower Carbohydrate fruits and veggies. This will lower your body's amount of sugar. Most of us are carb overloaded in this increases estrogen in our body which does negatively affect the thyroid. Add more healthy fats like to help balance your hormones like: coconut oil, coconut milk, avocado, grass-fed beef, wild salmon, chia, flaxseeds, and hemp seeds

Fermented foods are awesome to the belly. They make your gut very happy and from what this book has taught you. A healthy gut is very important to a better digestion and your thyroids health!

Keeping your Blood Sugar in Check

Low GI (glycemic index)/ Low Carb diets are based on the principles of balancing your blood sugar. The reason for keeping your blood sugar in check is to not have your blood sugar and insulin levels to rise to fast and high. This roller coaster of blood sugar highs and lows will activate your stress hormones and are catabolic to our tissues including the gut lining, lungs and brain. Your body is in one of two states throughout the day. You're either in an anabolic state or a catabolic state. If your body is in a constant catabolic state the protective barriers will become worn down over time and it over activates the immune system creating chaos where the body gets confused and attacks itself and wasting away as is the case with Hashimoto's or basically any autoimmune condition. Three things also can contribute to a catabolic state. Not working out smart. Not eating the right food. Not getting enough rest. If you are in a catabolic state you take the change of your body cannibalizing muscle. If you're in an anabolic state is it means that you're exercising correctly, you're eating the right foods and you are getting plenty of rest. Remember you can be creating more cortisol to store in your mid-section by over exercising. You want to stimulate the metabolism, not annihilate it. The easiest way to balance blood sugar and remain in an anabolic state is to eliminate processed carbohydrates and sugar, plan meals around protein and healthy fats then load up your plate with low carb/low GI.

Many people underestimate the importance in which their diet can have a direct effect on their thyroid levels. Eating certain foods can affect how well your body is able to absorb vital nutrients. A hypothyroidism diet is unlikely to "cure" hypothyroidism but it will certainly help to will reduce your symptoms. Eating certain foods and/or certain drinks (e.g. coffee) along with your medication can interfere with how your body reacts to the absorption and subsequently can change your thyroid levels. Most people with hypothyroidism are nutrient deficient, chemically toxic, and have a cortisol overload. Eating more nutrient-dense foods, reducing sugar intake, avoiding soy, making your own cleaning chemicals and avoiding preservatives may prove beneficial for overall health. Feeding your body with nutrient dense foods provides significant benefit in thyroid function and your hormonal biomarkers. Hormones are these little chemical messengers that are produced in one part of the body and released into the blood to trigger or regulate particular functions in other parts of your body. Your endocrine system is the supervisor. It's in charge of these network of glands throughout the body that regulate certain body functions, including body temperature, metabolism, growth, and sexual development. Understand that there are things that individually help to halter your thyroid ability to absorb your medication and you need specific foods to improve thyroid function. Our thyroid plays a most important role in metabolism. Along with your insulin and cortisol levels, thyroid hormones are an accelerating force behind metabolic rate and weight management. Many health problems start to appear if our thyroid stops working properly. Diet alone won't cure your hypothyroidism. Improving your dietary consumption by eating food that feed and heal your thyroid may also enhance T4 and T3 levels.

Why should I care about eating to cater to my thyroid or just eating healthy at all? Why all have to die someday.

Sometimes I want to shake people and say "Wake up!" You have to power to make a difference. You've always had the power. No one can force you to eat processed foods. Eating healthy isn't easy. Adjusting your life and catering to your specific health needs will benefit you in the long run. This is one of the smartest decisions that you can make. Not only will you start to look and feel better but think of the medical costs that you could be saving your future self. Not having the right nourishment makes your body sluggish, exhausted, and week. No one but you can do this. You have to be your own health advocate. Do you ever wonder what are the reasons why people are getting sick are? What is the real reason? Could it be pollution? Could it be radiation from cellular devices? Could it be global warming? Could it be lack of nutrients in our farming soil or pesticides in our food? Could it be the sneaky hidden sugars in our foods along with the saturated fat, extra sodium and tons of empty calories we consume mindlessly? No wonder our bodies are sick. The nutrients in food allow the cells in our bodies to perform their necessary functions. In other words, nutrients give our bodies instructions about how to function.

Here is a list of the top 4 causes of death in the United States. This is a statistic report from 2007 taken from the National Vital Statistics Report. None of these things may affect you directly but I am sure you know someone who it has. These numbers should scare you. You could be next.

There were total of 2,423,712 reported deaths in the United States in 2007.

1. Diseases of heart (heart disease)- 616,067 – 25.4 % of total deaths in 2007

2. Malignant neoplasms (cancer) – 562,875 – 23.2 % of total deaths in 2007

3. Cerebrovascular diseases (stroke) – 135,952

4. Chronic lower respiratory diseases – 127,924

EVERY CELL IN YOUR BODY CAN BE IMPACTED BY THYROID MALFUNCTION

Is eating to cater to your thyroid safe for your children?

Yes, real food is for everyone – children, teens and reluctant spouses. Helping your family switch from a modern American diet to nutritious, whole foods is one of the greatest gifts you can give them.

Why is gluten unhealthy?

Gluten is a component of all barley, wheat, and rye products. Eating gluten can increase in inflammation, which in turn disrupts function of the hypothalamic pituitary thyroid axis (HPTA). Disruption of the hypothalamic pituitary thyroid axis decreases conversion of T4 to T3, in return changing the absorption of thyroid hormones. People have found that their thyroid function improves upon the removal of gluten from their diets.

The truth about the good fats

Healthy fats: If your diet is lacking in healthy fats, you may want to consider increasing your consumption. One of the best ways to ensure that you're getting enough fat in your diet is to eat more avocados.

Avocados contain mostly monounsaturated fat and some polyunsaturated fat.

Avocados

Coconut oil

Dark chocolate

Eggs

Grass-fed butter

Nuts & Seeds

Eating more saturated fats also provides more benefits to those of us with hypothyroidism. Particularly, addition of unrefined, virgin coconut oil to the diet of individuals with hypothyroidism may: decrease brain fog, enhance cognitive performance, and boost overall physical energy. Coconut oil contains MCTs such as caprylic acid that modulate: blood sugar and metabolism, improve digestion, and reduce inflammatory responses.

Transitioning your Hypothyroidism family

Reluctant spouses, kids and teenagers

An easy way to get your kids excited about their new food journey is to involve them in the process. Encourage them to help you in the kitchen – younger children can do basic tasks like washing the vegetables; older kids can help chop, peel, and clean up. Teenagers can even be in charge of the family's dinner for one night. This is a great way to teach them how to start cooking real food. Also ask your kids what they would like to eat and have them help plan the weekly meals. You can even involve them in your grocery store trip where they can add their input and help you pick out the ingredients.

You want to provide your family with all the micronutrients they need to support a healthy growing body. Raising a healthy family has its own challenges, but it's not impossible, and the healthy eating habits your children learn will help guide them for the rest of their lives. Start off slowly with introducing a recipe or a hypothyroidism friendly snack. Slow and steady wins the race.

Tips to Make Your Family Dinner less Stressful

Tips to make dinner stress free

Most of us has hit our peak time of exhaustion by late afternoon. It's a roller coaster ride of craziness. You have so much to do in the a little bit of time. After work you have game practices, errands to run, car pools, extra-curricular activities and not to mention helping your child with homework. Cooking dinner seems like another daunting task added to your already busy life.

Recent research at Columbia University found that children who regularly had dinner with their families are less likely to abuse drugs or alcohol, and more likely to do better in school. In fact, studies show the best-adjusted children are those who eat with an adult at least five times a week, says Ann Von Berber, PhD, chair of the department of nutrition sciences at Texas Christian University in Fort Worth.

Organize in the a.m.

Try to wash and chop your vegetables ahead of time and store them in a Ziploc® brand Bag with a dry paper towel to absorb the moisture.

Assign dinner Duties

Make an after school chore chart where your kids know and can go straight to their after school tasks. Let them know that they are appreciated and the home couldn't manage without them doing their 'special" chore. It might not seem like much but setting the table is a big deal and it is certainly one less step to take.

Onions and garlic, oh my!

Onion or garlic sautéed with olive oil can add a delicious boost any dish. If you have a recipe that needs chopped garlic or onion try to pre chop or precook it. Place them in the freezer in a Ziploc® brand Freezer Bag for safe keeping until you need it.

Snack Time

Always try to give your kids a small healthy snack while you are cooking dinner. This will help to avoid you kids getting to fussy and irritated due to being hungry before dinner.

Hanging Out

It's always fun to hang out with your family and ask them how their day has gone while you are preparing the meal and this will run into dinner time. This is a good way to stay connected in our fast pace world. This will make you family feel closer and happier when you share about each other's day. Family mealtimes are a way to increase the time you spend talking with each other and most importantly being heard in a fast paced world.

Turn up the Tunes

You can turn on some good music while you are preparing the meal. This will start making memories with you children and everyone can enjoy the music. This also can let them know that the day is over with and it's okay to start to unwind.

Slow Cooker Needed

Don't let you slow cooker just sit in that cabinet! Slow cookers are awesome little cooking machines. Who doesn't like coming home to a cooked hot meal? All you have to do is wash up and plate your food. If you need slow cooker recipes. **My book A Survivors Guide to Kicking Hypothyroidisms Booty: The Slow Cooker Way has over 101 easy slow cooker recipes.**

Make Ahead Meals

Prep all your meals the week on Sunday. Place them in the freezer or fridge. Where all you have to do is grab the pre prepped ingredients when you come home and start cooking. This can save you 30 minutes of dinner prep time. Always use your judgement and follow food safety practices.

Hypothyroidism in times of illness

What to do if your family is feeling sick?

Bone Broth. The new green Juice?

Today across America there a new hot trend of beverages filling cups. So what is this new magical elixir? It's Bone broth. Bone broth is loaded full of minerals and nutrients that improve your gut and digestive system. This magical elixir has been considered a great healer in many cups across the world. You have to drink high quality bone broth that is made from humanely-raised, grass-fed cows and pasture raised chickens can help start to repair the lining of the gut.

Here are 6 reasons why you should try drinking bone broth.

1. Heal and seal your gut. According to Jill Grunewald, a holistic nutrition coach and founder of Healthful Elements, a cup a day works miracles for leaky gut syndrome but it's also good for protecting non-leaky guts. The gelatin in the bone broth (found in the knuckles, feet, and other joints) helps seal up holes in intestines. This helps cure chronic diarrhea, constipation, and even some food intolerances.

2. Protecting your joints. Bone broth has glucosamine and chondroitin in it. Glucosamine has been taking as a supplement for years. Bone broth has a ton of other benefits that will make your joints happy health and pain free.

3. Better Skin. Bone broth has a rich source of collagen. Today in a world full of body imaging procedures you will see a many products with collagen. It's a cheaper to just drink bone broth with collagen and start make your skin, hair, and nails look radiant naturally from foods.

4. Mood enhancer. Several studies have shown the glycine in bone broth has improved sleeping and memory functions.

5. Immune Booster. Mark Sisson, author of The Primal Blueprint, actually calls bone broth a "superfood" thanks to the high concentration of minerals. He says that the bone marrow can help strengthen your immune system. (Something that won't surprise your grandma who always made you her famous chicken soup when you got sick!) A Harvard study even showed that some people with auto-immune disorders experienced a relief of symptoms when drinking bone broth, with some achieving a complete remission.

6. Healthier bones. Bone broth is loaded with phosphorus, magnesium, and calcium which is an essential building blocks for healthier bones.

Chicken and Beef Broth

Ingredients:

(You don't have to use both sets of bones you can use one or the other)

4 lbs. chicken bones (any combination of backs, necks, and feet)

2 lbs. beef bones (shin or neck)

2 small onions, peeled and quartered

4 small carrots, cut into 1-inch pieces

4 stalks celery, cut into 1-inch pieces

1/2 bunch flat-leaf parsley

1 bunch fresh thyme

12 oz. can tomatoes, drained

1 head garlic, halved crosswise

1 tsp. black peppercorns

Directions:

Combine bones in a deep 8-quart pot.

Rinse with cold water, scrubbing with your hands.

Drain and pack bones in pot.

Cover with 4 inches of cold water and cook over medium-high heat for about 45 minutes until liquid boils.

Reduce heat to medium and move pot so burner is off to one side. (This helps broth to circulate.)

Simmer until broth looks clear, about 1 hour, occasionally using a ladle to skim off surface fats and foamy impurities.

When broth looks clear, add remaining ingredients and simmer for an additional 2 hours.

Use a spider skimmer to remove and discard bits of meat.

Put a fine-mesh strainer over another large pot and pour broth through it; discard solids.

Drink immediately, or let cool before storing. Makes 2 1/2 quarts.

Slow Cooker Simple Bone Broth

Ingredients

3-4 lbs. of bones

1 gallon water

2 tablespoons apple cider vinegar

Instructions

Add everything to the crockpot. Cook on low setting in crockpot for 10 hours. Cool the broth, strain and pour broth into container. Store in refrigerator. Scoop out the congealed fat on top of the broth. Heat broth when needed (with spices, vegetables, etc.).

Gut-Healing Vegetable Broth Recipe

This is a nutritious, gut-healing broth as a vegan alternative to bone broth.

Serves: 8

12 cups filtered water

1 tbsp. coconut oil or extra-virgin olive oil

1 red onion, quartered (with skins)

1 garlic bulb, smashed

1 chili pepper, roughly chopped (with seeds)

1 knob ginger, roughly chopped (with skin)

1 cup greens such as kale or spinach

3-4 cup mixed chopped vegetables and peelings (I used carrot peelings, red cabbage, fresh mushrooms, leeks and celery)

½ cup dried shiitake mushrooms

30g dried wakame seaweed

1 tbsp. peppercorns

2 tbsp. ground turmeric

1 tbsp. coconut aminos*

A bunch of fresh coriander or other herb of your choice (plus extra, to serve)

(Optional) ¼ cup nutritional yeast, for extra flavor and vitamins

Instructions

Simply add everything to a large pot. Bring to a boil then simmer, with the lid on, for about an hour.

Once everything has been cooked down, strain the liquid into a large bowl.

Serve immediately with some fresh herbs, for decoration or cool for later. It also freezes well.

Vegan Bone Broth Alternative

This version contains lots of nutritional goodness that is great for overall health but particularly focuses on plenty of gut-healing properties.

The main stars are:

Wakame seaweed: Great source of omega 3 – one of the best for vegans, great for intestinal health, full of vitamins and minerals (particularly good source of iron, calcium, magnesium and iodine). Not suitable for SCD diets, leave out as necessary.

Shiitake mushrooms: Gives the most amazing, comforting flavor. Full of vitamins and minerals (great source of vitamin D – especially if sun dried, zinc and B vitamins). Contains all essential amino acids. Prebiotic.

Coconut oil or olive oil: Healthy fats with a good omega ratio that help absorb nutrients.

Turmeric: Powerful anti-inflammatory plus adds delicious flavor and a beautiful color.

Spinach or kale: Full of vitamins and minerals (particularly high in Vitamins K, A and C, magnesium and calcium). Also a good source of protein and omega 3. Prebiotic.

Coconut aminos: Mainly used for flavor but also gives the benefit of its amino acids. May not be suitable for some diets as it's considered a sugar, so leave out if necessary.

One cannot think well, love well, and sleep well if one has not dined well.

—*Virginia Woolf 1882-1941, A Room of One's Own*

About the recipes

All of these recipes are catered towards healing your thyroid. You won't find any recipes with cruciferous vegetables in this book. Although cruciferous vegetables are excellent for your health it has been proven to interfere with thyroid function when eaten raw. Please limit your cooked cruciferous vegetable intake to 2x a week until you get your thyroid working at the optimum level again. Cruciferous vegetables are rich sources of sulfur-containing compounds known as glucosinolates. Some glucosinolates found in raw cruciferous vegetables produces a compound known as goitrin, which has been found to interfere with thyroid hormone poduction. Very high intakes of raw cruciferous vegetables, such as raw cabbage and raw turnips, have been found to cause hypothyroidism. The reason for this book is give you the tools you need so you're not in the kitchen cooking 3 different meals. All the recipes are nutrient packed to supply your thyroid with the help is needs to support your thyroid plus everyone will enjoy them. Your family will think you're a master in the kitchen! People with hypothyroidism may feel that they have a limited selection of foods but you don't! Remember food is information. It's more than just calories. The type of food you eat will determine if you're to be healthy or sick. You must tailor your nutritional needs to your body. Being on a very restrictive diet when you don't to be can put you at risk for adrenal fatigue and nutrient deficiencies.

A diet for hypothyroidism should include whole foods rich in iodine: whole baked organic potatoes with skin, cod, dried seaweed, shrimp, Himalayan crystal salt, baked turkey breast, dried prunes, navy beans, tuna, boiled eggs, lobster, cranberries, and green beans. Niacin-rich foods (required for normal manufacture of thyroid hormone) are tuna, chicken, prunes, bananas, turkey, salmon, sardines, and brown rice.

Riboflavin-rich foods:

Raw almonds, eggs, mushrooms, sesame seeds, salmon, and tuna.

Zinc: (as well as vitamins B6, C, and E, iodine) is a major component of thyroid hormone balance and is antimicrobial. Zinc-rich foods (boost thyroid function) are white cooked button mushrooms, chickpeas, kidney beans, dark chocolate (70 percent or higher), pumpkin, squash seeds, and almonds.

Selenium-rich foods: (helps to convert T-4 to T-3) are Brazil nuts and tuna.

High-polyphenols foods: (acts as an anti-fungal) are cocoa powder, dark chocolate, coffee, tea, flaxseed meal, red raspberries, blueberries, black currants.

Vitamin B6–rich foods: (required for normal manufacture of thyroid hormone) are raw unsalted sunflower seeds, quinoa, raw pumpkin seeds, sesame seeds, flaxseeds, pistachio nuts, cashews, tuna, halibut, salmon, dried prunes, bananas, avocados, dried apricots, and raisins.

Vitamin C–rich foods: (boost thyroid gland function) are bell peppers, dark leafy greens, kiwis, broccoli, berries, citrus fruits, tomatoes, peas, and papayas.

Riboflavin-rich foods: (or vitamin b2—essential for normal manufacture of thyroid hormone) are frozen peas, beets, crimini mushrooms, eggs, asparagus, almonds, and turkey.

Vitamin E–rich foods: (work with zinc and vitamin A to produce thyroid hormone) are raw almonds, shrimp, avocados, quinoa, salmon, extra-virgin olive oil, and cooked butternut squash.

See you are NOT limited to what you can eat with hypothyroidism. You have many options to what you can eat and why you need to be eating this. Here are more foods and YES you may read repeats from the paragraph above but I want you to see what an abundance of foods that you can eat. The only limit you have in the kitchen is your imagination. My recipes are a starting point. You can start to creating your favorite recipes and healing your thyroid as you eat! Your diet is part of the solution.

Fatty fish like wild salmon, trout, halibut, cod, albacore tuna, flounder, cod or sardines (omega-3s and selenium) only a few times per week….

No farmed fish, period!

No gluten.

Split peas, lentils, black beans, kidney beans, pinto beans, artichokes, raspberries, blackberries, chia seeds, red apples with skin, prunes, green peas, raw almonds, garbanzo beans, winter squash, spaghetti squash, summer squash, butternut squash, zucchini, popcorn (no microwave-ready, bagged popcorn), cherries, citrus fruits, kiwi, cantaloupe, papaya, mango, plums and red grapes, tomatoes, carrots, gluten-free, steel-cut oats or gluten-free rolled oats, watermelon, green tea, organic apple cider vinegar, lemon, garlic, leeks, parsley, celery, ginger root, tomatoes, cucumbers, carrots, asparagus, organic whole baked potatoes with skin, shrimp, Himalayan crystal salt, Celtic sea salt, baked turkey breast, dried prunes, navy beans, gluten free steel cut or rolled oats, cranberries and green beans, organic no hormone chicken, brown rice, raw almonds, eggs, sesame seeds,, chickpeas, kidney beans, dark chocolate 70 percent or higher, walnuts, cocoa powder, hempseeds, red raspberries, blueberries, black currants, brazil nuts, raw unsalted sunflower seeds, quinoa, raw pumpkin seeds, sesame seeds, flaxseeds, pistachio nuts, cashews, dried prunes, bananas, avocados, dried apricots, and raisins, red, green and orange bell peppers, romaine lettuce, kiwis, papayas, beets, all mushrooms, quinoa, extra-virgin olive oil and cooked butter nut squash. sea vegetables, dried seaweed, kelp, dulse, nori, arame, wakame, kombu, tomato paste, brewer's yeast, brown rice, algae, healing spices (Ceylon cinnamon, turmeric, gloves, cayenne pepper, garlic, oregano, sage, ginger .

Hypothyroidism at Social Functions

Hypothyroidism tricks and tip for attending a party or gathering

Macadamia Coconut Balls

2 cups unsweetened shredded coconut

1/3 cup macadamia nuts

1 banana

1/2 tsp vanilla extract

1 Tbsp. maple syrup

1 Tbsp. melted coconut oil

A pinch of nutmeg

In a food processor, process 1 cup of the coconut and all of the macadamia nuts. Add your coconut oil and pulse 10 seconds. In a medium-sized bowl, peel and mash your banana. Next add the vanilla extract, maple syrup, and nutmeg. Place the mixture from the food processor to the bowl and mix well. Using your hands, roll the mixture into one or two inch balls. Scoop up the remaining shredded coconut and pat onto each ball, coating it thoroughly. Keep your balls in the refrigerator in an air-tight container.

Fire Roasted Tomato Salsa with Cilantro and Lime

2 cans (14.5 oz. each) Any Organic Fire Roasted Diced Tomatoes, well drained

1 medium onion, chopped

2 cloves garlic, finely chopped

1/4 cup chopped fresh cilantro

1 tablespoon fresh lime juice

1/2 teaspoon coarse salt (kosher or sea salt)

1 to 2 fresh jalapeño seeded, finely chopped

In medium bowl, stir together all ingredients. Serve with Gluten free chips.

Zesty Pico

1 cup avocado, skin removed and cut into ½ chunks

1 1/4 cups coarsely chopped fresh tomato

3 tablespoons chopped onion

1/2 clove garlic, minced

1 tablespoon sliced jalapeño pepper, seeds removed

3 tablespoons fresh chopped cilantro

1/4   teaspoon salt

2 tablespoons fresh lime juice

Smash your avocado until it is the chunkiness that you desire. Next add the rest of the ingredients. Mix well to combine all ingredients in a bowl. You can use tortilla chips, pita chips and sliced fresh vegetables such as cucumber, carrot, bell pepper, celery and zucchini to dip.

Mediterranean Hummus

2 1/2   cups low-sodium canned garbanzos, drained

1/2   cup water

1/2   cup tahini

6 tablespoons fresh lemon juice

4 garlic cloves, or to taste

1/2 teaspoon Himalayan sea salt

2 teaspoons onion powder

Combine all ingredients in a food process or blender. Blend on high 1–2 minutes until smooth and creamy. Chill in a covered container before serving. You can use tortilla chips, pita chips and sliced fresh vegetables such as cucumber, carrot, bell pepper, celery and zucchini to dip.

Vine Ripened Bruschetta

2/3 cup canned low-sodium cannellini beans, drained and rinsed

5 tomatoes washed, rinsed and diced

2 tablespoons extra-virgin olive oil

3 tablespoons sun-dried tomatoes in oil, drained and finely chopped

3 cloves garlic, minced

2 tablespoons fresh rosemary, chopped

Mix all the ingredients in the olive oil. Let it sit for 30 minutes to blend the flavors. Serve on our bruschetta bread.

Cranberry Quinoa almond Butter Power Bars

2 Cups of cooked quinoa

2 Cups of gluten free uncooked oats

1/2 Cups of dried cranberries

1/2 Cups of smooth almond nut butter

1/2 Cups of almond milk

1/3 Cup of raw honey

1/4 Cup of ground flaxseed

1 tsp Ceylon cinnamon

Follow the directions and cook you quinoa as directed on the package. Preheat your oven to 350. Combine all the ingredients in a bowl together and stir until everything is mixed well.

Place in a 7x11 baking pan. Cook in the oven for 12-15 minutes.

Beyond the food: The Hypothyroidism Lifestyle

Stress:

Stress weakens our body causing to break down and allows you to be more susceptible to illness. You can have control over your lifestyle, thoughts, emotions, and stress. One of main things you can start to do is realize the sources of your stress. Sometimes we all feel like there's nothing we can do about the stress. The bills won't stop coming, there will never be more hours in the day, and your work and family responsibilities will always be demanding. That's just life. You do have the power and you can take the control over your stress. Keep in mind there isn't a "one size fits all" solution to managing stress and we all respond differently to it. I am here to let you know that you can take action and here are a few things you can do for stress management. There is a better and healthier way to cope. You can go for a walk, call a friend, take your pet for a walk, take a hot bubble bath with Epsom salt, plant a garden, listen to music, watch a funny movie, get lost in a good book, drink some chamomile tea. Another thing you can start to do is keep a stress journal which will help you identify the regular stressors in your life and the way you deal with them. Each time you feel stressed, keep track of it in your journal. As you keep a daily log, you will begin to see patterns and common themes. In your journal write down:

- What happened to make you stress
- How it made you feel, both physically and emotionally
- How you responded to it
- How you made yourself feel better

Stress relieving foods. Organic blueberries, 70% dark chocolate, wild salmon, avocado, pistachios, leafy greens, turkey, seeds, oatmeal and sunshine.

Stress causing foods. Sugar, gluten and processed foods.

Write yourself a gratitude list. Don't just list what you have. List why you appreciate what you have. Embellish them, bask in them, and be specific to why you appreciate it. Be grateful for small mercies. Only when you live life with eyes of gratitude that you can truly see the world for what it is. Gratitude is an attitude that has a lot of benefits.

Goats Milk Stress Bath Reliever

2 cups of powdered goat's milk

2 cup of Epsom salt

1 cup of sea salt

2 cup of baking soda

10 drops of lavender essential oil

Combine the dry ingredients and the lavender essential oil. Store in a closed container. When you are ready to take a bath, add 1 cup of dry ingredients. (Kids can use up to 1/2 cup of the mixture.) Bathe 3 times weekly, soaking for at least 12 minutes.

Epsom salt is rich in magnesium and sulfate in which are easily absorbed through the skin. Many of us are deficient in magnesium and we don't even know it. Magnesium is the second most abundant element in our cells, helps to regulate our bodies 325 enzymes, and plays an important role in organizing many bodily functions, like muscle control, electrical impulses, energy production, and the elimination of harmful toxins.

According to the National Academy of Sciences, American's magnesium deficiency helps to account for high rates of heart disease, stroke, osteoporosis, arthritis and joint pain, digestive maladies, stress-related illnesses, chronic fatigue and a number of other ailments.

(You want more body recipes? You can find them in my book: Awareness has Magic)

Exercise:

Technology has made our lives simply easier. People are not as active because frankly they don't have to be. People use to have to walk to work and walk to the grocery store and just basically walk to get to anywhere they needed to be. Our modern age has given us cars to drive and machines to wash our clothes. We seem to enjoy entertainment in front of a TV or computer screen. The local grocery store have made it more convenient to purchase produce than to plant a garden. Not to mention how easy it is in our fast paced, stressed out world to run through a drive thru to grab dinner instead of slaving over a hot stove. We are burning off less calories and eating more high fat, less nutrient based foods. Exercise is very important part of staying healthy. It helps you lose weight, boost your confidence, release feel-good chemicals into your body called endorphins, reduces PMS symptoms, boost your sex drive, is a natural antidepressant, boost your self-confidence, it can help you sleep better, strengthens muscles and bones and lower the risk of some diseases. It doesn't matter what your current weight is. When you are being active it boosts high-density lipoprotein (HDL), or "good," cholesterol and decreases unhealthy triglycerides. Physical activity stimulates those brain chemicals that may leave you feeling happier and less stressed. In return, you will feel better about your appearance and this will boost your confidence and improve your self-esteem. Regular physical activity shouldn't just be based on losing weight or what you currently weigh. I want you to start to get active in your own way. One of the biggest reasons people stop exercising is they get bored with it, no support, or motivation. Try to switch it up, change your routine and have fun with it. You can start to do little things like park further away, take the stairs, take up dancing at your local community center, join a Zumba group, use your push mower, and find a partner to walk with or go window shopping. Try keeping you music playlist fresh and up to beat, set realistic goals, talk about your work out on your media platform, like Facebook, Instagram, and twitter or in Sunday school class. You can also add some competition and challenge a friend. The Bottom Line is If you get bored walking on the treadmill or in your exercise class, then stop doing what you don't like and find something that truly arouses you. Fall in love with the challenge of physical living, instead of chasing after the results of becoming fit. Take responsibility for your own enjoyment. Don't forget one major rule: It must involve some sort of spirited movement!

Body Care:

The Environmental Working Group evaluated over 72,000 products and ranked them in an easy-to-understand guide to make sure you have a resource to keep your family safe. Check out EWG's "Skin Deep Cosmetic Database" today @ http://www.ewg.org/skindeep/. You have to start reading labels and avoiding conventional body care products that are high in DEA, parabens, propylene glycol and sodium lauryl sulfate these products are full of toxins. Plastic bottles should be replaced with glass and stainless steel due to the toxic effects of BPA. Also, change your cookware from Teflon pans to stainless steel, ceramic or cast iron this will start make a big difference in your thyroid health.

All natural hair lightener Recipe #1

½ cup raw honey

½ cup extra virgin olive oil

½ banana, smashed

Mix everything in a jar. Allow to sit for 1 hour then apply to your hair. Wrap your hair in a plastic grocery bag than wrap with a towel. This will lock in the heat. Allow the mixture to sit on your hair for 1-2 hours. The honey works as a natural high lightener. It has a peroxide affect.

All natural hair lightener recipe #2

¼ cup honey

½ cup conditioner

Mix everything in a jar. Mix everything in a jar. Allow to sit for 1 hour then apply to your hair. Wrap your hair in a plastic grocery bag than wrap with a towel. This will lock in the heat. Allow the mixture to sit on your hair for 1-2 hours. The honey works as a natural high lightener. It has a peroxide affect.

All natural hair lightener recipe #3

10 bags of chamomile tea

4 lemons

2 cups of boiling water

1 spray bottle

Boil your water in a small pot. Pour your hot water in a glass safe container. Place the tea bags in the water. Allow them to sit for 10 minutes. Take a spoon or fork and press the tea to the side of the jar to ensure you get all the chamomile tea. Next squeeze the juice of the four lemons in the container. Allow the mixture to cool enough to be safe to pour in your spray bottle. Spray the mixture on your hair as you sit out in the sun and allow your hair to dry.

All natural hair lightener recipe #4

2 tablespoons of raw honey

2 tablespoons of cinnamon

¼ cup of water

1 tablespoon of extra virgin olive oil

Mix all the ingredients and allow to sit for 1 hour. Apply to your hair. Wrap your hair in a plastic grocery bag than wrap with a towel. This will lock in the heat. Allow the mixture to sit on your hair for 1-2 hours and then rinse out. You can apply this twice a week until you get the desired results.

Homemade all natural shampoo

2/3 cup of castile soap

Two teaspoons of almond or olive oil

10 drops of your favorite food grade essential oil

½ cup of coconut milk

Mix all the ingredients in a bottle. Use when needed.

Natural remedies to cure a yeast infection:

First thing is you must do is stop eating all bad carbs and sugars. Yeast feed off of bad carbs and sugars!

1. You can take an organic tampon dip it in organic yogurt no additives and insert change every 2-4 hours for 48 hours increase water intake.

2. You can take an organic tampon soak it in a diluted mixture of 20/80 Braggs apple cider vinegar with the 20 being the vinegar and 80 being purified water

3. You can freeze organic yogurt in Popsicle molds and insert in your vagina to melt while you sleep.

4. At bed time you can insert a probiotic and allow it to dissolve over night while you sleep.

5. You can douche with Kefir and add an extra probiotic for an extra punch

6. Douche with a 50/50 mixture of food grade hydrogen peroxide and purified water

7. If the lips to your vagina are itchy and irritated, apply organic coconut oil to soothe.

8. Take a baking soda bath. An entire small box of baking soda to your warm water. Sit with your legs open & rotate, move, splash the water towards your "area". Do this for about 30 minutes. Think of it as "marinating" your stuff so to speak.

9. Make sure your orally taking a probiotic

10. Start eating fermented foods

11. Drink organic cranberry juice

12. You can freeze into Popsicle molds a 50/50 mixture of organic coconut oil and yogurt. Insert at night allow it to melt while you sleep.

Eliminating Toxic House Hold Cleaners

Did you know that the products you clean your house with can cause a hormonal imbalance?

Many chemicals used in commercial cleaning products are known to have negative effects on our endocrine system. Many of these chemicals are linked to hormonal disruption and they also effect the nervous system, irritate your eyes, your skin and your airway. These harmful store bought Household cleaning products get into your system when you are using them when you breathe them in or get them on your skin where they are easily absorbed. When you use laundry detergents, fabric softeners and dryer sheets, the chemicals they contain often stay on your clothes, where they can be absorbed easily through your skin. You know that great smell after mopping the floor or cleaning that shower? Well, those chemicals leave a residue that evaporates and lingers around the home as it "off gases" throughout the day. According the Environmental Protection Agency, indoor pollution can be up to 100 times higher than outdoors, in part because of chemicals in household cleaning products. This is why you should learn to make your own cleaning products!

If you don't want to make your own cleaning products. The Environmental Working Group evaluated over 72,000 products and ranked them in an easy-to-understand guide to make sure you have a resource to keep your family safe. Check out EWG's "Skin Deep Cosmetic Database" today @ http://www.ewg.org/skindeep/

Here are few non-toxic cleaners that you can make out of your very own kitchen! If you would like more recipes please pick up my book: The Survivors Cookbook Guide to Kicking Hypothyroidism's Booty.

Readers are urged to all appropriate precautions before taking on any do-it-yourself task. Always follow the directions and use precautions when making your own homemade products. Never stretch your abilities too far. Each individual, fabric, or material may react differently to particular suggested use. Although this is a nontoxic and natural way to clean your home, always wear protective gloves and eyewear. Although every effort has been made to provide you with the best possible information, neither the publisher nor author are responsible for accidents, injuries, damage incurred as a result of tasks performed by readers. The author will not assume responsibility for personal or property damages from resulting in the use of formulas found in this book. This book is not a substitute for professional services.

Natural All-Purpose Floor Cleaner

2 cup distilled vinegar

2 cups water

4 cups of water

4 tablespoons of washing soda

Mix the washing soda with 4 cups of water in a bucket. Dampen you mop with the mixture. Mop well. Next, rinse mop with regular water. Pour out mixture, rinse bucket, and place regular water in the bucket and go over the mopped area. Next, place the 2 cups of vinegar and 2 cups of water mixture in a bucket and dampen the mop. Mop well.

The Tipsy Lavender-and-Lemon Bathroom Disinfecting Spray

1/2 cup white vinegar

1/2 cup vodka

10 drops lavender essential oil

10 drops lemon essential oil

1 1/2 cups water

Fill your bottle with water; add your drops of lavender and lemon essential oils. Next, add your vodka and white vinegar. Mix well. Spray on your bathroom surfaces and let sit for 10–30 minutes. Wipe off with a no microbial cloth. Don't forget to label your spray bottle with a black permanent marker.

Natural Oven Cleaner

1 ¼ cup of baking soda

¼ cup of vinegar

10 drop soft lemon food grade essential oil

2 teaspoons of liquid Castile soap

Half a cup of natural salt.

Mix the ingredients with a quarter cup of water, then put into a plastic spray bottle. Also worth trying – put a few drops of dish soap on half a lemon and use it to scrub.

Natural Furniture Polish

1 cup of Olive oil

½ of a freshly squeezed lemon

1 bowl

1 cloth

Mix both ingredients into the bowl and allow the cloth. Wipe your furniture with the cloth.

Shower Cleaner Formula

1 Teaspoon of dish soap.

1 Teaspoon of dishwasher rinse aid

1/2 a cup of food grade hydrogen peroxide.

½ cup of alcohol.

Pour each ingredient in a spray bottle. Shake well to mix. Spray on your shower and allow to sit for 10 minutes before scrubbing. Rinse and repeat if needed.

Homemade Granite Cleaner

1/4 teaspoon of liquid dish soap

1/4 cup of rubbing alcohol

2 1/2 cups of water

Pour all the ingredients in a spray bottle and shake to mix. Spray on your granite counter and make sure you rinse it well with a clean cloth with only water on it.

Carpet Stain Remover

1 cup of water

1 cup of vinegar

Mix the ingredients in a spray bottle and spray on the carpet stain. Allow to sit for a few minutes and carefully dab up.

Heavy Duty Carpet Cleaner

1/4 cup of salt

¼ cup of vinegar

1/4 cup of borax

Mix well and rub into the carpet in a circular motion. Use clean water to help wipe the mixture away.

Home Made Windex

1/4 Cup (4oz) Isopropyl Rubbing Alcohol

Pour the alcohol into a spray bottle and spray on your window. Wipe clean with a cloth.

Home-Made Febreze

¼ cup water

20 drops of your favorite essential oil

Place in a plastic spray bottle, fill the remaining space with hot water and give it a shake.

Toilet Cleaner

10 drops of Lavender Essential Oil

10 drops of Tea Tree Oi.

1/3 cup of white vinegar

1/3 cup of baking soda

Place the baking soda in the toilet, next add your drops of essential oils and finally pour in your vinegar. Allow to sit for 20 minutes next scrub the mixture and flush.

Natural Bleach Alternative

6 cups water

1/4 cup fresh lemon juice

1 cup of food grade hydrogen peroxide

Pour the mixture in a safe container to store in your laundry room. You can add ½-1 whole cup per load and this can be used as a household cleaner.

Natural Disinfectant Cleaning Wipes Alternative

1/4 cup of vinegar

1 cup of water

10 drops of eucalyptus essential oil

10 drops of lemon essential oil

7 drops of tea tree essential oil

Mix the solution in a spray bottle. Spray on the surface of what you want disinfected and wipe clean with some old cut up clothes.

You can burn White Sage Smudge Sticks. This herb that cleanses, purifies and heals the body. By burning white sage, you can expect to see and smell white smoke billowing out from it creating a festive and herbal delight.

Stovetop Potpourri

Ingredients:

2 cups fresh cranberries

3 tangerines, halved

3 whole cinnamon sticks

2 star anise

1 teaspoon whole cloves

1 vanilla bean + 1 tablespoon vanilla extract

1 small branch fresh pine

1 cup pomegranate

Water

Combine all ingredients in pot, filling 3/4 of the pot with water. Bring to boil, then turn down heat and allow to simmer for at least 4 hours. Continue to add water to the pot, as the liquid evaporates. You can let the pot cool down overnight, and reheat and simmer the next day, for a full weekend of Christmas goodness.

Crock Pot Simmer

1 orange sliced

2 cups of water

2 tablespoon of vanilla extract

4 cinnamon sticks

Combine all ingredients in your crockpot and allow to slowly cook on low. Your house will smell amazing. You can also make this recipe on the stove.

Homemade Potpourri

Ingredients

Cloves

Cinnamon sticks

Star anise

Oranges

Apples

Pine cones

Instructions

1. Preheat oven to 250 degrees. Slice apples and oranges thin, really thin. Place in a single layer on cookie sheets and bake for an hour and a half, check every half hour thereafter. Once dry, mix with your spices. Jar and allow to "marinate" for a day. Place this in a bowl to make your house smell fantastic!

Natural Room deodorizer

1 cup of coffee grounds

Place you coffee grounds in a bowl, cup or container with a lid that has holes in the top. The coffee will absorb orders. Replace and throw away often.

Natural Room Freshener

Your favorite essential oil

(Rosemary, vanilla and lemon is a nice smelling combo)

Cotton balls

Small container

Place a cotton ball in a small container and add 15 drops of your favorite essential oil. Place this around your home. Also, every time you replace your air filter, add 10-15 drops of your favorite essential oil and this will make your entire house smell good. You can also place a few drops on a light bulb.

Homemade Air Freshener

Small Mason Jars

Cloth

Baking soda

Essential oil

Fill your mason jar half way with baking soda. Add 15 drops of your favorite essential oils. Lay the fabric across the lid of the jar and place the ring of the jar to seal it. You want the fabric just big enough to be able to seal the jar and cut a few slits in the cloth.

All natural Room Spray

This non-toxic alternative will have your home smelling great in no time!

10-20 drops of your favorite Essential oils

1 clean spray bottle 16 oz. of distilled water

Pour the water in your spray bottle and then add your essential oil.

Store in dark, cool place and shake it before use. You can spray on furniture, linens or in the air to refresh your home.

Natural Carpet Cleaner

Baking Soda

Sprinkle baking soda on any carpet and allow to sit 20 minutes. Vacuum the baking soda up and it will help release dirt and orders from your carpet.

Grease Cutting floor cleaner

1/4 cup vinegar

1 tablespoon of dawn dish soap

¼ cup washing soda

Add your ingredients to a bucket that is half way full of water. Once you blend it, it will become full of bubbles. It does go away and dry very well.

Shower and Tub Cleaner

Spray bottle

1 cup of vinegar

1 cup of dawn dish detergent

You want equal amounts of each. Pour in your spray bottle and label it. Spray on your shower or tub and allow it to sit for 1 hour then proceed to scrub the area and rinse well.

This homemade laundry detergent recipe not only keeps those harsh chemicals away, but it's also cheaper, lasts longer, and made with all-natural ingredients; it's a greener, healthier alternative to commercial chemically loaded products. There's nothing more natural or better than natural products like vinegar, baking soda, and essential oils.

Homemade Powder Laundry Soap

I mix mine in a large bucket then pour it in a large glass container with a 1/4 small scoop. Only 3 ingredients to make this detergent! Add 3 cups each of the washing soda and borax detergent booster. Mix well. Grate one bar of FELS-NAPTHA soap in a bowl. (Any castile soap or ivory soap will work too.) All you need is 1/4 of a cup for each load, and this is exactly the scoop size that I use. Makes things easier for me. Your laundry will be fresh, clean, and actually smell good.

Vinegar of the Four Thieves Insect Repellent Ingredients****

- 1 32 ounce bottle of Apple Cider Vinegar
- 2 TBSP each of dried Sage, Rosemary, Lavender, Thyme and Mint
- At least quart size glass jar with airtight lid

How to Make the Vinegar of the Four Thieves Insect Repellent

Pour your vinegar and dried herbs into large glass jar. Seal it tightly and store it in a place where you can see it daily to shake it for 2 weeks. After 2 weeks, strain the herbs out and store in spray bottles and keep in the fridge. When you use it on your skin, dilute to half with water in a spray bottle and use as needed.

All natural wasps trap

1/4 cup vinegar

1/2 cup of warm water

1/2 cup sugar

1 teaspoon salt

Mix this solution in an open container, place where needed. Make sure it is out of the hands of children. Although it's nontoxic they might still be able to get stunk if they put their hands in the container.

How can I lose weight?

It seemed no matter what diet I tried, I couldn't lose the weight. No matter what exercise I tried, I couldn't shed the weight. What I was missing and what I didn't figure out until much later is that there were many things at play with my weight loss battle. The thyroid medication that I was taking was synthetic T4. I needed my T3 to be converted as well. See, my T3 was my energy hormone and I suffered from this horrible imbalance of my T4 not converting to T3 which lead to my adrenal fatigue. My system was so over worked, I had a lack of nutrients and my body was severely imbalanced. The adrenal fatigue put my body in a battle and my cortisol levels were out of this world! Cortisol add fat around my mid-section. So, the harder I exercised, the more "cortisol"-fat added to my stomach. Then let's mention the leaky gut. My gut played a vital role in my autoimmunity. 95% of all thyroid diseases are autoimmune. Most often undiagnosed. I needed to get my gut fixed. The only way I was going to start to put my Hashimoto's in remission is to start working on my gut. The 70% of my immune system is manufactured in my gut. Like an onion, I started to work on each layer that needed to be addressed, peeling it back, layer by layer. Did I have food sensitives? Many people have food sensitives continue to eat these foods that causes a leaky gut, candida and ph imbalances. Gluten, dairy, soy, eggs and processed foods are just a few. Also, no matter how much I worked on my foods and exercise. It wasn't going do me any good if I continued to use household cleaners, under arm deodorants and fluoride toothpastes. The list can go on and one. I needed to start reading labels and not allow these toxins on my body. I was fighting an uphill battle for my life. I started by the elimination process. Uncovered what foods bothered me, fixed my gut, slowed down my exercise and switched my medication to Armour. I started eating clean, fermented veggies, low carb and healthy high fat. Reading food labels, if it was artificial or made in a lab I avoided it. If I couldn't eat it, I didn't put it on my body. I avoided all environmental toxins like the plague. I added vital vitamins and minerals that my body was missing and probiotics. This was my secret to my success to my weight loss.

I added more things like:

Olives

- Avocado
- Cooked Cruciferous vegetables (Limit this to no more than 2x per week)
- Fermented foods
- Fatty fish (e.g., wild-caught salmon trout, tuna and mackerel.)
- Chicken and Turkey (organic hormone & Antibiotic free)
- Grass Fed Beef
- leafy greens
- Nitrate free bacon
- Nuts, such as walnuts and almonds
- Seeds, such as pumpkin, chia and flax
- Coconut Flour, Almond Flour and hemp seeds
- Chia Seeds
- Kelp and seaweed
- Celtic or Himalayan sea salt

- coconut
- coconut oil
- organic butter (preferably Grass fed)
- ghee
- Bone Broth
- Eggs: Look for pastured or omega-3 whole eggs. (if you don't have a food allergy)
- Cheese: Unprocessed cheese (cheddar, goat, cream, blue or mozzarella).
- Fish oil (EPA/DHA)
- Magnesium
- Vitamin B Complex
- Vitamin C
- Vitamin D3
- Zinc
- Ancient Nutrition- Bone Broth Collagen Loaded with Bone Broth Co-Factors

Do you have weight loss tunnel vision syndrome?

How to look at your weight loss vision.

When you picked up this book, I hope that losing weight wasn't your main goal. Of course, we all have that picture perfect imagine that we want to see when we look in the mirror. For some strange reason we think that our lives would be so much easier, if we could just be "that" size. If we could wear those shorts or that cute little strapless top without feeling like an escaped circus freak act. Losing weight could also mean extending your life, getting off certain medications, seeing your grandkids grown up. Whatever your REAL reasons are for losing weight it is an added benefit but being the healthiest you is the ultimate goal. Some of us get weight loss tunnel vision. We are so focused on the scale and our weekly weight loss "drama" that it will make you miserable and start to stress you more out where you become your own worst enemy. Emotional eating, here I come! This isn't about you losing weight. It is about you reaching your goals. Stop allowing yourself to fall back in your old ways. This is a journey. Don't focus on the scale. Focus on your weight loss vision. Focus on your health.

Is your Hypothyroidism Self Sabotaging your Workouts?

We all know that regular exercise is an important part of your overall health. Exercise burns calories to prevent weight gain and helps speed up your metabolism. It is also a releases endorphins to give you those mood-enhancing chemicals. What if I told you that exercise can cause adrenal crashes due to your already high cortisol issues? You could be stressing your thyroid out even more and not even realizing it. Are you exercising but not getting any results? Are you still gaining weight, feeling constantly fatigued, irritable and moody and often battling some other sort of sickness? You could be actually stressing your body more out by over-exercising.

The magic word here is cortisol.

Cortisol, a steroid hormone produced by the adrenal gland. It is released in response to stress. When you are stressed, your body releases certain "fight-or-flight" stress hormones that are produced in the adrenal glands: cortisol, norepinephrine and epinephrine. Staying stressed raises your cortisol levels and your body actually resists weight loss. Your body thinks times are hard and you might starve, so it hoards the fat you eat or what you have presently on your body. Cortisol will grab fat from your butt and hips, and move it to your abdomen which has more cortisol receptors. Hello there Mrs. Muffin Top!

Today most of us are in a chronic stress state. However, our body doesn't know the difference between car troubles, relationship issues, debt, work pressure and truly life-threatening stress. This is why our body is still ready to defend and will react exactly the same as it always has done.

Over-exercising can:

- Deplete hormones necessary for the functioning of the body
- Cause gradual bone loss
- Increase injuries
- Cause cramping of muscles
- Add to inflammation
- Increase healing time
- Affect cardiac function

Affect blood flow

Decrease the ability of muscles to use fatty acids as a source of energy

Reduce endurance

Here are a few things you can start to change in your life:

1. Limit your caffeine to 200 milligrams a day. (This is equal to about one 12 oz. cup of coffee)

2. Start eating a true Keto diet. Yes, there are other fantastic suggestions on what you need to eat but in doing so you will avoid simple carbs, processed foods, and refined grains, and get plenty of high-quality protein, healthy fats and great organic low GI/Low Carb vegetables. It will get you started. You need to fight this inflammation that is raging in your body. Atkins and Keto are two different things. Although they may be similar in some ways but completely different.

3. It is okay to say NO! Take time to relax, take a nap, distress and recuperate.

4. Start building your endurance back slowly.

5. Get a heart rate monitor and use it. Know your heart rate comfort zone.

6. Listen to your body. How do you feel the next day? Do you need an extra day to recover?

7. Set realistic goals, one step at a time and don't get discouraged.

8. Try a Low-impact aerobics workout. Something to get your heart rate up and your lungs pumping without putting too much stress on your joints, which is important because joint pain is another common symptom of hypothyroidism.

9. Strength training is good. Strength training builds muscle mass, and muscle burns more calories than fat, even when you're at rest.

10. Get some sleep!

Just think how great it's going to feel when you are as healthy on the inside as you look on the outside! The ultimate goal isn't to look fit but to be fit.

Did You Know That Your Body Has its Very Own Personal Food Code?

There is so much information overload that most women are confused as to where to start to begin creating a healthy lifestyle balance. Perhaps one of the biggest misconceptions is the ambivalence of it all. We all get super busy in this thing called life. Sometimes we lose a little piece of ourselves traveling back in fourth.

How many times this week have you said to yourself, "If my life wasn't so busy, I would be able to start exercising" or" Why did I eat that extra cookie?" or" its 3a.m., why can't I sleep?!" Or" Why am I so exhausted?"

Frankly, life is one big tug a war between feeling completely insane to the creativity at it all.

Why do we allow ourselves to become Stressed Out, Overwhelmed, and Totally Exhausted and continue to carry around those extra ungodly pounds that we dreadfully despise? After 5 years of carrying that excess weight, I am here to tell you, from one female to another, you can't technically call it baby weight gain any longer.

Have you ever wondered why people respond differently to losing weight?

In the last fifty years what has changed in our society? We have the same predisposition genetics as our grandparents. We are unique and come in all different shapes, sizes, race, religions and greed.

We can't blame is all on genetics being unhealthy solely on the DNA that was passed down to us. Everyone's genetic makeup is different. It's like your fingerprints.

In school, I was always that girl who was tall, skinny, freckled faced, wavy blonde hair with a flat chest and a flat butt. I remember being plagued at school for being too skinny. Having no shape. Tormented about my freckles. While other school mates were well endowed with large boobs, hippy hips and a nice rounder booty. Our metabolisms certainly dictate how we use energy and our genetics can dictate how we are shaped but what has started to interests me more-so lately is why we store fat on certain areas of our bodies when others don't.

These questions have confused and frustrated people and health care practitioners for decades. But why is it so confusing? One thing we have learned is each of us are unique and have our very own biochemistry that sets us apart from everyone else. Although we might share the same common traits and perhaps the same overlapping metabolic tendencies. We can't continue to say that one-size-fits-all when it comes to our very own unique body chemistry. There are over 7 billion people on this planet and we come in all different shapes, colors and sizes. With this being said wouldn't you think the one-size-fits-all- approach to losing weight wouldn't work since we are we are all unique. With this all being said wouldn't you think that we all have our very own personal food code too?

Finding Your Food Code

Finding your food code won't be as easy as it sounds. Quite frankly you will have to put some elbow grease into this but it's not unattainable. How we live from day to day is completely different on every spectrum across the board. One thing I do know for-sure is that every single day no matter who we are or where we live our bodies are bombarded with a toxic burden of chemicals, we are not feeding our bodies the proper nutrients, we are nutritional deficient, and some of us have little to no activity & these are some of the reasons why our bodies are becoming stagnant and increasingly polluted. It would be silly to take Motrin for a pebble stuck in your shoe when all you had to do was pluck it out. So why not on this journey go ahead, do some research and start addressing the issues at hand.

We are creating a perfect storm within our bodies. The less nutrients we consume, more toxins we add, create this world win of health issues. It's sad that our western diet is made up of red meats, vegetable oils, white flour and sugar. Who would of thought that something so simple as eating has become so complicated. Food does matter. It talks to your DNA. Food can change your DNA!

The foods you eat have a major impact your life — It affects your gut health and along with increasing or decreasing the inflammation in your body. Unfortunately, our western world diet are full of foods that have a bad impact on both your gut and your inflammation. If it was made in a lab, avoid it. Do a little research and you will find that our western diet that is made up of processed, fake foods, chemicals, sugar and corn oils are all highly flaming the fan of your inflammation.

We have a shortage of nutrients in our food system. The most common foods that you load up your grocery cart with are loaded with bad carbs, fillers, preservatives, additives, flavorings, and chemicals. Your body doesn't have any idea what do to with all this fake food. We are creating a weaker human race, inflammation and pain along with the possibility of welcoming other diseases and disorders. Your diet and lifestyle choices is what has caused any health issues that you may have unless you were born with a health issue then you can look at your parents diet , surroundings and lifestyle choices. It can go back generations. The only way to get back our health and vitality is to look at the root of it all.

You can change and control your life.

Think about what you're putting in your body. Either you're fighting disease or feeding disease. You must get a concept of nutrient density. Gluten, dairy and soy products create inflammation in the digestive tract. In ancient times grains were prepared by soaking, sprouting and fermenting but that tradition in making them been long forgotten with our fast-paced culture.

Let's talk more about store bought bread:

The bread you're buying at the store really isn't real bread you're buying. The white bread in the grocery is not the bread that our ancestors use to eat. 65% of the foods we eat are made from grains that are grown in a field such as grain bread, whiskey pasta and beer just to name a few. Wheat is made up of 3 parts the bran, the germ and the starchy endosperm.

The way the grain is processed has a huge impact not only on the way it taste and how healthy it is for you. Our ancestors used every part of the grain when they made their bread. White bread on the store shelves is made by an industrial process that strips out the wheat into all-purpose flour and in most cases if you read the back of the labels you will see chemicals additives added. These chemical additives is what gives white bread a longer shelve life.

White bread is also only made from the starchy endosperm which your body turns into pure sugar.

If you have inflammation in the digestive system undigested proteins leak into the blood stream creating a heightened immune reaction that often can lead to a leaky gut which causes other problems.

Most often than none, it's unrealistic for any lifestyle change to happen overnight. It does take practice but with practice does come change. Don't allow the bigger picture to discourage you. Every small thing you change to better your health will pay off in the end. It's the small steps that can make a big difference. Start by looking at your life and evaluating the toxins you may regularly come in contact with, understand what must take priority, and replace with these alternative options that I have listed in this article.

You have the power to make a difference in your life. You've always had the power. No one can force you to become more aware of what you put on your body and what you put in your body. What you eat is just as important as what you put on your body. Adjusting your life, reading labels and catering to your specific health needs isn't easy but it will benefit you in the long run. This is one of the smartest decisions that you can make. Not only will you start to look and feel better but think of the medical cost that you could be saving your future self.

Healthy Cells Grow From the Inside Out

Look into getting a Knowledgeable Holistic Health Practitioner:

The very first thing that you need to do is look into getting a knowledgeable holistic health practitioner!

The main reason why you should work with a knowledgeable health practitioner is its patient-centered medical healing at its best. Unfortunately, when it comes to your body there isn't a one size fits all approach to dealing with it and often times you are left still searching for the answers to your symptoms when all you want is your zest for life back. A knowledgeable health practitioner will care for you as a individual as they won't look at your body as a whole they will treat each individual body symptom, imbalance and dysfunction. They will take into consideration the whole person, including physical, mental and spiritual aspects, when treating a health condition or promoting wellness. I want you to understand that you are made up of interdependent parts and if one part is not working properly, all the other parts will be affected. A knowledgeable health practitioner certainly moves from the confusion of the "one size fits all treatment" approach that we know isn't working to the one that will cater to what your body needs. Let's not forget that each of us are a unique case and unless you get a proper thorough clinical evaluation, trying to figure what medical advise you need online is dubious at best.

In order to find your food code here are a list of things that need to be addressed in your life. When all these things are addressed and you are learning to know what your body needs and needs to avoid then you can find your personal food code. I never said it was going to be easy.

1. Address Food sensitivities

Food allergies

Many people are unaware that certain foods are actually working against their bodies. You should see a specialist and be tested to ensure you have no food allergies. Your lymphatic system can also be affected by your gut. If your gut is inflamed and not healed this is taxing on your immune system which in return is taxing on your lymphatic system. Consider adding prebiotics and probiotics to help support gut health along with eating properly and avoiding these common food allergens.

Common food allergens that can contribute to an inflamed gut are:

Nightshades

Eggs

Grains (gluten)

Dairy

Legumes

If you allergic to certain foods it is will involve you're the immune system. You know that your immune system controls how your body defends itself. Your body see's inflammatory foods as invaders and will kick in your autoimmunity responses. For example if you have a food allergy to cow's milk, your immune system will see cow's milk as an invader. In-return your immune system overreacts by producing antibodies called Immunoglobulin E (IgE). These antibodies travel to cells that release chemicals, causing an allergic reaction to start fighting for your body. Being tested for food allergies seems to be easiest way to check to see if you have any food allergies so you can start avoiding these foods and help your immune system become strong again.

2. Address nutritional deficiencies

Having nutritional deficiencies certainly adds gas to the fire. When you are deficient it can aggravate the symptoms: vitamin D, iron, omega-3 fatty acids, selenium, zinc, copper, vitamin A, the B vitamins, and iodine.

3. Address Chronic Candida

Did you know that an overload of Candida was picked up at birth or shortly thereafter? We were supposed to be getting good friendly bacteria from our mother's at birth, but "our" mother's had Candida overgrowth and unknowing passed it on to us. And over the years, our bodies has become more and more compromised. Your gut microbes could be dramatically affecting your thyroid health. There is a lot of misinformation and misunderstanding about Candida. Both from the medical profession and on the internet. It is easy to get fooled into thinking, as many sites will try to convince you, that all anyone needs to do is to take their product or buy their e-book. Of course, they will all have testimonies. What they don't tell you in those testimonies is how the Candida came back — in a month or two or in six months. However long it took for the

Candida to overgrow enough to start causing symptoms again. It is important to know that dealing with Candida is not an easy fix.

4. Address Hormonal imbalances

After researching many hours on this topic, I've found that where your body stores fat is hint to what is going on with you internally with your hormones. As our hormone levels change with age, pregnancy, exercise, eating habits, or other life events, fat adjusts itself to our every changing hormonal events and places itself in different area's in our body. Our hormones have a direct impact on how much body fat we store and where it is stored on our bodies. Wouldn't it be wonderful to know what approach to take to fix those thunder thighs or that muffin top? Now even with this information its just a stepping stone of knowledge to better equip you a healthier you. This completely changes how you and what you should be eating.

So what exactly does it mean to have fat stored in certain areas of your body and not others?

Love handles/belly: Love handles often means that you are way too stressed out and when you're stressed out it raises your cortisol levels. It could also be an indicator that you might have adrenal fatigue. Cortisol adds fat around my mid-section.

You are eating too much sugar where you become insulin resistant. If your body is in constant elevated levels of insulin (a hormone that regulates the metabolism of carbohydrates in the bloodstream) it will accumulate around your mid-section. A lack of sleep also may lead to metabolic issues and help encourage those love handles. It also could mean you have elevated estrogen levels and more insulin production. So what do you need to do? Stop eating crap, those processed carbs and avoid sugar, even the fake sugars which are even more horrible for you. You should also go easy on the exercise, sometimes if you exercise more it adds more cortisol to your body so you are fighting a losing battle, try yoga, more sleep, meditation, Pilates, planks, lifting weights and walking are good ways to start. Don't forget fat gained around the waist is dangerous in terms of it increases the risk of heart disease, diabetes and other chronic diseases.

Thighs: Sometimes it's our genetic bone structure that was passed down from our parents that gives us more hips or fatter thighs than the next person and other times it can mean that we have elevated estrogen levels. This is the female sex hormone. Thigh fat is a little harder to burn off than belly fat. You can also have fluid retention in your thighs. So many think that fluid retention only takes place only in the abdomen but that isn't true It actually occurs all over your body. So what do you need to do? Start drinking your daily needed allowance of water. Your body weight and divide it by two. That's the least amount of water to drink per day and please don't drink it all in one sitting. There is a think called water toxicity and it will kill you. Space out your water consumption. Choose better skin care products in my blog 21 Successful Tips on Clean Beauty Swaps. I share with your skin care products are healthier. You want to avoid chemicals such as BPA (that can be found in plastic containers, water bottles and pretty much anything plastic unless it states BPA FREE), parabens or phthalates. Your food should be 100% organic and you most defiantly should be avoiding all soy products like the black plague. Let's not forget that getting in a good night's sleep will also help to improve your estrogen levels.

Back of Arms: This could mean that you have lower testosterone levels as well as an excess insulin. Women do have a small amount of testosterone in our adrenal glands and ovaries although this is thought as a male hormone. Start eating more avocados, as in healthy fats and fatty fish such as salmon can help improve this area. Try to avoid all red meat and all dairy products. Start trying to lift some weights. Building muscle through weight lifting can and may also increase testosterone levels.

Upper Back: This could mean you have lower levels of Thyroxine and higher levels of insulin. Thyroxine is a thyroid hormone that plays a role with your metabolism and calorie burning rate and this hormone is secreted into our bloodstream. You can help boost your thyroxine naturally by eating foods such as shellfish, seafood and cruciferous vegetables, avoiding gluten and soy, and increasing healthy fat intake.

Our metabolism does not decide to burn or store body fat based on calories. It makes these decisions based on the hormones those calories trigger. That is why the quality of calories matters so much….higher-quality calories trigger body-fat-burning hormones while low-quality calories trigger body-fat-storing hormones.

Body fat is important necessity for life. It is our source of energy and it stores some much needed nutrients, a major ingredient in brain tissue. Moreover, it provides a padding to protect internal organs and insulates the body against the cold. But yet, getting too fat (more than 30 percent body fat in females and 25 percent in males) can be dangerous and is associated with increased risk of disease and premature death, regardless of where the fat is stored in the body. As a American society, we are tipping the scales to the point that obesity is now a national health epidemic.

Here are some other factors that contribute to estrogen dominance:

Eating clean. Let's talk about eating clean whole nutrient rich foods. Start reading label. If you must eat prepacked foods always look for foods that have a short ingredient list and things that are recognizable as actual food. Various chemicals are added like sugars, questionable oils, and sodium and so on. Always avoid soy and if soy is listed as an ingredient. Soy comes in all varieties and are highly processed, high in refined starches, heated oils and again added sugar, salt and low in nutrients and fiber. Oh let's not fail to mention that soy mimics your hormones and plays a very sneaky trick on your endocrine system.

Poultry or beef raised on hormones. Although it may cost a little bit extra try to eat free-range or grass-fed animals that are raised without hormones and antibiotics.

Chemicals found in consumer products Personal care products loaded with parabens, petroleum, and phthalates. Did you know that products we use every day may contain toxic chemicals and has been linked to women's health issues? They are hidden endocrine disruptors and are very tricky chemicals that play havoc on our bodies. "We are all routinely exposed to endocrine disruptors, and this has the potential to significantly harm the health of our youth," said Renee Sharp, EWG's director of research. "It's important to do what we can to avoid them, but at the same time we can't shop our way out of the problem. We need to have a real chemical policy reform." The longer the length of ingredients on your food label means how much more unhealthy it is for you to consume. When an item contains a host of ingredients that most likely you cant even pronounce or remember to spell you can bet your lucky dollar that the natural nutrients are long gone. These highly processed frank n foods are very difficult for the body to break down and some of the chemicals will become stored in your body. Click on this link to see what you should avoid.

You can also find many great DIY personal care recipes alternatives in my book, AWARENESS HAS MAGIC. Here are three recipes from my book **AWARENESS HAS MAGIC.**

Lemon Cream Body Butter

6 Tablespoons coconut oil

¼ cup cocoa butter

1 Tablespoon vitamin E oil

3 drops of Lemon essential oil or 3 drops of your favorite essential oil

Over low heat in a double boiler, put the coconut oil and cocoa butter in a bowl. When it has almost completely melted, remove from the heat and add the vitamin E oil and essential oil. Allow the mixture to cool until it solidifies. Lastly mix the body butter vigorously with a spatula, and then transfer it to a mason jar with a sealable lid. Date and label your product. If you don't care for the lemon essential oil, use whatever smells best to you. This is your journey not mine I am only here to help guide you.

Homemade Shaving Cream

1 cup shea butter

1 cup virgin coconut oil

3 Tablespoons vitamin E oil

3 Tablespoons sweet almond oil or olive oil or jojoba oil

3 Tablespoons Dr. Bonners Liquid Castile Soap

30 drops of lavender essential oil (optional)

30 drops of lemon essential oil (optional)

I like to use an electric mixer, mixing all ingredients until stiff peaks are formed (approximately 2-3 minutes). Store in a mason jar with a sealable lid.

Mosquito Repellent

15 drops of lavender

4 tbsp. of vanilla extract

1/4 cup freshly squeezed lemon juice

Place all these ingredients in a 16oz then fill with water.

Insomnia. It's amazing how the food we eat affects our health, sleep patterns and even our "gasp" sex drives. Unfortunately, when you don't get enough sleep, it can age us faster , cause depression, weight gain, make us forget things, gives us headaches and we have a greater chance of developing heart disease. If you have issues like snoring or sleep apnea and are overweight, one thing you can do is lower your body fat index. For those of us that don't have snoring or sleep apnea we ask the question," Sleep why you hate me so much!" We need to feed our bodies to get more, Tryptophan, serotonin and melatonin. (serotonin is a brain chemical that helps you sleep) and melatonin (the hormone that makes you sleepy) Trytophan is an essential amino acid, which means you have to gt it from your diet because your body cannot produce it.Your body uses tryptophan to make the neurotransmitters serotonin and melatonin. Red Onion Teahelps with insomniaDirections

1 cup of water

1 onion, cut in quarters

Blend, strain and drink

Epsom salt bath which is rich in magnesium

Sleepy time Goats Milk Bath

2 cups of powdered goat's milk

2 cup of Epsom salt

1 cup of sea salt

2 cup of baking soda

10 drops of lavender essential oil

Combine the dry ingredients and the lavender essential oil. Store in a closed container. When you are ready to take a bath add 1 cup of dry ingredients. (Kids can use up to 1/2 cup of the mixture). Bathe 3 times weekly, soaking for at least 12 minutes.

Lavender has a reputation as a mild tranquilizer. Simply dab a bit of the oil onto your temples and forehead before you hit the pillow. The aroma should help send you off to sleep.

Lastly, don't obsess over not sleeping. Studies have shown that people who worry about falling asleep have greater trouble falling asleep! It may help to remind yourself that while sleeplessness is a pain in the ass it isn't life-threatening. Let's try to be mellow-bellow. Eat foods that foods contribute to calmness and sleepiness.

5 plants to help you sleep better!

1. Aloe Vera — emits oxygen at night to help you combat insomnia and improve the overall sleep quality.

2. Lavender- Lavender is a plant that is well known to induce sleep and reduce anxiety. The smell of lavender slows down your heart rate and reduces anxiety levels.

3. Jasmine plant- The smell of jasmine has been shown to improve the quality of sleep.

4. English Ivy- it's beneficial for those who have breathing problems and asthma. Studies have shown that English ivy can reduce air molds to 94% in 12 hours.

5. Snake plant- emits oxygen into the night while you sleep, taking carbon dioxide from the air inside your home. It also filters nasty household toxins from the home.

Poor liver function due to the use of pharmaceuticals drugs. You really need to do research on your medications. Some medications have a negative effect on your lymph system and since estrogen is metabolized primarily in the liver try to not use pharmaceutical drugs unless absolutely necessary. If you must take these medications then try introducing liver-supporting supplements into your diet, such as cucumber juice, milk thistle extract, calcium d-glucarate, folic acid and taurine.https://www.lymphnet.org/membersOnly/dl/reprint/Vol_24/Vol_24-N4_Drugs_LE.pdf

Magnesium deficiencies: Magnesium is necessary for metabolizing estrogen in the liver. Magnesium is a mineral that plays a important part in our health and well-being. It's one of the forgotten minerals and it's vital for many processes within the body. Magnesium helps to keep the nervous system healthy and to calm your nerves when you are stressed. In fact, did you know that magnesium is the first mineral depleted when you are stressed? So if you have any type of stress in your life magnesium is the first mineral that goes out the window. Magnesium is also an important mineral co-factor for enzymes that have biochemical reactions in the body. In other words it plays a large role in digestive system health as it helps enzymes do their job as well as to loosen the body to relax and ease to support the metabolic processes. These recipes are from my book AWARENESS HAS MAGIC.

Calming Magnesium Body Butter My homemade magnesium body butter will help replace the magnesium that our bodies need to thrive to survive. I always try to apply a little to my feet and shoulders before bed. This helps me relax and also get a fantastic night's sleep. It's pretty easy to make and the benefits are overwhelming. Magnesium deficiency is very common and it mimics other common symptoms and many other conditions like, being tired and felling run down, not sleeping well, getting headaches, gut issues, and even feeling stressed and anxious. Here is a list of things that can lower our magnesium levels:

- Too much caffeine
- Processed food and Sugar
- Too much stress
- Poor sleep habits

Calming Magnesium Body Butter

1/2 cup cocoa butter

1/2 cup of coconut oil and melt

1/4 cup magnesium oil

Add 10 drops of lavender essential oil,

Add 10 drops cedarwood essential oil

Add 10 drops frankincense essential oil

Place a heat-safe glass measuring cup/bowl inside a pot that has 1-2 inches of simmering water over medium heat. Add the cocoa butter and melt it in your double boiler until it's completely melted.

Remove the cocoa butter from heat, and add 1/2 cup extra virgin coconut oil to the melted cocoa butter and stir until completely the coconut oil has melted. Next add 1/4 cup magnesium oil to the mixture and combine. Place the mixture in the refrigerator to cool for about 30-60 minutes (until it is cooled completely). After the mixture has completely cooled and became a solid. Use a hand mixer or stand mixer to whip it. Start on low and increase speed slowly. Whip for about 3-5 minutes. Next add the 10 drops each of lavender essential oil, the 10 drops of cedar wood essential oil, and the 10 drops of frankincense essential oil. Scrape down the sides of the bowl and continue whipping for another 5 minutes or so, until the magnesium body butter is light and fluffy. The color of the magnesium body butter will change from yellow to a pale ivory and almost white color. Lastly put the magnesium body butter into mason jars and seal tightly with a lid. Make sure to label and date the top of the lid. This recipe makes enough for two 4 oz. glass jars.

Household chemicals: Did you know that it takes 26 seconds for the chemicals to enter into your bloodstream? The real reality is we are damaging our DNA and we are changing our genetic makeup for future generations. There was a study a few years back that said the umbilical cord of an average American baby has over 200 known chemicals in it. Eighty percent of the common chemicals that are used daily in this country, we know almost nothing about. Our children are being born toxic and we have no idea if these toxins are already doing some sort of damage their brains, their immune system, their reproductive system, and any other developing organs. Are we unknowingly setting ourselves up for failure in the womb, even before birth?

Scientists and researchers are concerned that many of these chemicals may be carcinogenic or wreak havoc with our hormones, our body's regulating system.

Most products have a warning label that is typed in bold "Keep out of Reach of Children". As consumers, we believe that if our children don't ingest these products they will not be harmed by them. This can be far from the truth. Think about other common methods of exposure are through the skin and our respiratory tract. WE are along with our children are often in contact with the chemical residues housecleaning products do leave behind, by crawling, lying and sitting on the freshly cleaned floor.

Scientists at Norway's University of Bergen tracked 6,000 people, with an average age of 34 at the time of enrollment in the study, who used the cleaning products over a period of two decades, according to the research published in the American Thoracic Society's American Journal of Respiratory and Critical Care Medicine.

These chemicals can chemicals bind together.

Exposure to phthalates has been associated with lower IQ levels.

These chemicals can also be found in the shampoos, conditioners, body sprays, hair sprays, perfumes, make up, cleaning supplies, colognes, soap and nail polish that we use.

The results follow a study by French scientists in September 2017 that found nurses who used disinfectants to clean surfaces at least once a week had a 24 percent to 32 percent increased risk of developing lung disease.

Scientists and researchers are concerned that many of these chemicals may be carcinogenic or wreak havoc with our hormones, our body's regulating system.

It's not enough to be aware of all the outdoor chemicals that we are exposed to everyday but inside our homes we can have more power and control. We have to be more aware about using chemical cleaners, paints, glues, body lotions, toothpastes, underarm deodorants, hair products and pesticides. Instead start to begin to use products that don't pollute our very own bodies. We must read labels, make our own products and do our own research. I can't stress this enough. We must take a stand for our health. Stop using commercial products that are laced with unknown and harmful body damaging products.

You can reduce your exposure to them by eating organic foods, making your own cleaning chemicals and using alternative pest control methods.

You can also find many great recipes for alternative cleaning solutions in my book **AWARENESS HAS MAGIC.**

Here are two recipes from my book **AWARENESS HAS MAGIC.**

Vanilla grapefruit linen spray

2-1/2 cups filtered water

3 drops pink grapefruit essential oil

2 drops vanilla essential oil

1/4 cup vodka

The vodka helps the water dry quickly after you spray it on your linens. Theses essential oils that are used create a beautifully fresh vanilla grapefruit scent that is perfect for a summer pick me up. This spray is very versatile. It can be used on clothing, fabric furniture, or even as a quick air freshener.

If the vodka smell is slightly strong just add another drop or two of essential oil.

Always shake the bottle be before spraying on your linen.

Tub & Tile Cleaner

1/4 cup baking soda

1/4 cup lemon juice

Or 10 drops of lemon essential oil

3 Tablespoons Epsom salt

3 Tablespoons Sal Suds or Castile liquid soap

1/2 cup white vinegar

Pour the vinegar into the bottle, followed by the baking soda and Epsom salt. Shake the bottle to combine the ingredients. Add the Sal suds gently shaking the bottle to combine. Mix all ingredients in a bottle with a sealable lid.

Scrub and then rinse with water and wet clean rag.

5. Parasites and Heavy Metals

   Heavy metals weaken our body's defense system against foreign invaders and make it convenient for them to set up house. American's are not being protected as we should from pollution. We don't have to go to a 3rd world country or even a foreign country be subjected to contaminated water which can led to illnesses. The pollution in our air, water, food supply, cleaning products, body products, commercial weed killers and chem trails in our environment. It's really hard not to have some sort of health issues that come from a heavy metal over load on our bodies. Just imagine commercial meat production, can goods and prepackaged foods. Heavy metals make a very acid environment which is very harmful to your gut flora where parasites and candida love to flourish. Candida and parasites actually do serve a purpose in your body they are to protect us from the potentially fatal complications of heavy metal poisoning. They feed on heavy metals and store them within biofilms- buffering us from heavy metal overload.

   Do you find that you are developing new allergies as you become older; are you always tired, do you have poor digestion, gas, heartburn; sugar cravings, are you irritable, frequent headaches; poor memory, "fogged in" feeling, dizziness, recurring depression, vaginal infections, menstrual difficulties, urinary tract infections, infertility, hay fever, postnasal drip, habitual coughing, catch colds easily, sore throat, athlete's foot, skin rash, psoriasis, cold extremities, arthritis-like symptoms, do you feel miserable in general? If answered yes to most of these symptoms then should be tested for candidiasis.

According to the publication in 1995 "Parasitic Diseases" it states the following rate of infection per species.

Nematodes (Round Worms)	1 billion individuals
Cestodes (Tape Worms)	300 million individuals
Tremadodes (Flukes)	300 million individuals
Protozoa (Amoebas)	1 billion individuals
Arthropods (Insects parasites)	500 million individuals

How can I start to detox from Parasites and Heavy Metals?

Each person is different and I encourage you to seek out a qualified nutritionist or other qualified healthcare practitioner in order to assess exactly which nutri-ents, herbs, homeopathic and nat-ural reme-dies and/or in which com-bi-na-tion that will help you achieve your goal. No one treatment is the same since we all have different diary needs, illness's and lift styles.

Getting the root cause of your issues are the main objective. I strongly recommend you get with your health care provider and allow them to schedule you for further tested if needed. This is how and where you will figure your own personal food code.

6. Heal your Gut

Your gut is your portal to health. It houses 80 percent of your immune system, and without your gut being healthy it is practically impossible to have a healthy immune system. A leaky gut have been linked to hormonal imbalances, autoimmune diseases such as rheumatoid arthritis and Hashimotos thyroiditis, diabetes, chronic fatigue, fibromyalgia, anxiety, depression, eczema and rosacea, and that is just to name a few. So you can understand why a properly working digestive system (your gut) is vital to your health. Contrary to what we use to believe. We now know that having a leaky gut is one of the main reasons, and probably the beginning stage, for developing an autoimmune disease. Having a leaky gut means that the tight junctions that usually hold the walls of your intestines together have become loose, allowing undigested food particles, microbes, toxins, and more to leave your gut and enter your bloodstream. This will cause your body to become full of inflammation, which in return will start to trigger an autoimmune condition and if you already have an autoimmune condition it will certainly make it worse. Luckily for you. Your gut is made up of wonderful cells that can turn over very quickly, so you can start to heal your gut in as little as thirty days, by following these 4 R guidelines: Remove, Restore, Replace and Repair

Remove the damage — Remove these inflammatory foods, household & body chemicals, drink filtered water(to avoid fluoride and chloride) , stop using aluminum brand deodorant, start using fluoride free brand tooth pastes, start to reduce your stress that damage your gut, do a detox to heal any gut infections from yeast, parasites, or bacteria.

Restore the Strong — replenish the enzymes and digestive acids that are necessary for proper digestion

Replace with friendly Bacteria — Make sure you are taking plenty a good strong probiotic that is full of these much needed "good bacteria" to start supporting your immune system. Here is a great product that I use. You can do your own research and I am sure there are other brands out there that are wonderful too. Garden Of Life Dr. Formulated Probiotics Once Daily Women's, 30 Count

Repair the digestive Tract — Give you gut a fighting chance by supplying the nutrients and amino acids needed to build a healthy gut lining. (Gelatin can improve your ability to produce adequate gastric acid secretions that are needed for proper digestion and nutrient absorption. Glycine from gelatin is important for restoring a healthy mucosal lining in the stomach and facilitating with the balance of digestive enzymes (Here is a brand that I use Garden of Life RAW Enzymes Women, 90 Capsules) and stomach acid. The best way to consume gelatin make them into broth or soup. You can do this by simply brewing some bone broth at home using this Bone Broth Recipe.

The real reality is we are damaging our DNA and we are changing our genetic makeup for future generations. There was a study a few years back that said the umbilical cord of an average American baby has over 200 known chemicals in it. Eighty percent of the common chemicals that are used daily in this country, we know almost nothing about. Our children are being born toxic and we have no idea if these toxins are already doing some sort of damage their brains, their immune system, their reproductive system, and any other developing organs. Are we unknowingly setting ourselves up for failure in the womb, even before birth?

Scientists and researchers are concerned that many of these chemicals may be carcinogenic or wreak havoc with our hormones, our body's regulating system. But the impact of these chemicals may be most severe on the developing brain, Perera said.

Brain development is the "most complete and most rapid during the first nine months, prenatally," she said. During that time, neural connections and pathways are being developed.

"Any interference by a physical stress like a toxic chemical or other stressor can disrupt this natural progression that is so very delicate and complex," explained Perera.

Though the group hopes to come up with regulatory recommendations to reduce this toxic burden, there are some simple things that individuals can do to reduce their exposure.

Children exposed to higher levels of these pesticides have been found to have higher rates of attention-deficit hyperactivity disorder.

Most products have a warning label that is typed in bold "Keep out of Reach of Children". As consumers, we believe that if our children don't ingest these products they will not be harmed by them. This can be far from the truth. Think about other common methods of exposure are through the skin and our respiratory tract. WE are along with our children are often in contact with the chemical residues housecleaning products do leave behind, by crawling, lying and sitting on the freshly cleaned floor.

Scientists at Norway's University of Bergen tracked 6,000 people, with an average age of 34 at the time of enrollment in the study, who used the cleaning products over a period of two decades, according to the research published in the American Thoracic Society's American Journal of Respiratory and Critical Care Medicine.

They found that lung function decline in women who regularly used the products, such as those who worked as cleaners, was equivalent over the period to those with a 20-cigarette daily smoking habit.

Everyday chemicals carry toxic burden

These chemicals can chemicals bind together.

Exposure to phthalates has been associated with lower IQ levels.

These chemicals can also be found in the shampoos, conditioners, body sprays, hair sprays, perfumes, make up, cleaning supplies, colognes, soap and nail polish that we use.

The results follow a study by French scientists in September 2017 that found nurses who used disinfectants to clean surfaces at least once a week had a 24 percent to 32 percent increased risk of developing lung disease.

 Scientists and researchers are concerned that many of these chemicals may be carcinogenic or wreak havoc with our hormones, our body's regulating system.

It's not enough to be aware of all the outdoor chemicals that we are exposed to everyday but inside our homes we can have more power and control. We have to be more aware about using chemical cleaners, paints, glues, body lotions, toothpastes, underarm deodorants, hair products and pesticides. Instead start to begin to use products that don't pollute our very own bodies. We must read labels, make our own products and do our own research. I can't stress this enough. We must take a stand for our health. Stop using commercial products that are laced with unknown and harmful body damaging products.

Did you know that products we use every day may contain toxic chemicals and has been linked to women's health issues? They are hidden endocrine disruptors and are very tricky chemicals that play havoc on our bodies. "We are all routinely exposed to endocrine disruptors, and this has the potential to significantly harm the health of our youth," said Renee Sharp, EWG's director of research. "It's important to do what we can to avoid them, but at the same time we can't shop our way out of the problem. We need to have a real chemical policy reform." The longer the length of ingredients on your food label means how much more unhealthy it is for you to consume. When an item contains a host of ingredients that most likely you cant even pronounce or remember to spell you can bet your lucky dollar that the natural nutrients are long gone. These highly processed frank n foods are very difficult for the body to break down and some of the chemicals will become stored in your body. Click on this link to see what you should avoid.

Pesticides, herbicides, GMOs in our food, fluoride and chlorine and trace pharmaceutical residue in the water supplies, methane, carbon monoxide and industrial pollutants in the air, and the toxic chemicals in our everyday household products.

No wonder our bodies are completely bombarded and overwhelmed with the constant exposed to toxic chemicals through the air that we breathe, the water we drink, the foods we eat, and the personal care products and cleaning products we use.

Every Cell in your body responds to the foods you eat, the products you put on your body to the house hold chemicals that you purchase for your home. All of these things have a direct impact on your hormones and in return your hormones have a direct impact on every major system in your body. Not to mention that our body is lacking certain nutrients that heavily influence the function of every cell in our body.

For starters, the three essential categories into which most of the hazardous ingredients in household cleaning products fall are:

1. Carcinogens– Carcinogens cause cancer and/or promote cancer's growth.

2. Endocrine disruptors – Endocrine disruptors mimic human hormones, confusing the body with false signals. Exposure to endocrine disruptors can lead to numerous health concerns including reproductive, developmental, growth and behavior problems. Endocrine disruptors have been linked to reduced fertility, premature puberty, miscarriage, menstrual problems, challenged immune systems, abnormal prostate size, ADHD, non-Hodgkin's lymphoma and certain cancers.

3. Neurotoxins – Neurotoxins alter neurons, affecting brain activity, causing a range of problems from headaches to loss of intellect

TAKING CUES FROM PRODUCT LABELS

You may find it time-consuming to research all of the ingredients in the cleaning products under the kitchen sink, in your garage or even in the bathroom but trust me. It is worth the hassle. Over all, product warning labels can be a useful first line of defense. These companies are required by law to include label warnings on their cleaning products if harmful ingredients are included. From safest to most dangerous, the warning signals are:

Signal Word

Toxicity if swallowed, inhaled or absorbed through the skin*

Caution

One ounce to a pint may be harmful or fatal

Warning

One teaspoon to one ounce may be harmful or fatal

Danger

One taste to one teaspoon is fatal

You can reduce your exposure to them by eating organic foods, making your own cleaning chemicals and using alternative pest control methods.

SALT

The Dietary Guidelines for Americans recommend limiting sodium to less than 2,300 mg a day—or 1,500 mg if you're age fifty-one or older or if you are black or if you have high blood pressure, diabetes, or chronic kidney disease. Read labels; it seems everything has sodium in it. Our bodies are on a sodium overload!

Pink Himalayan salt is naturally rich in iodine, so it doesn't need to be artificially added in. It also helps to create an electrolyte balance in your body, increases hydration, regulates water content both inside and outside of cells, balance pH (alkaline/acidity), and help to reduce acid reflux, prevents muscle cramping, aids in proper metabolism functioning, strengthen bones, lower blood pressure, help the intestines absorb nutrients, prevent goiters, improve circulation, dissolve and eliminate sediment to remove toxins. So, how much is 1,500 mg of salt? It is ¾ of a teaspoon.

Unbelievable!

Another thing many hypothyroid sufferers deal with is the lack of iodine in their body. Iodine is a critical essential trace element in our diet. Our bodies can't make iodine; therefore we have to rely on food to obtain it. This essential trace element is an absolute necessity for normal growth and development. In the year 1924, the Morton Salt Company, at the request of the government, historically started to add iodine to their salt mixture (in the form of potassium iodide). Table salt that you buy out of the store is bad for you anyway. "Table salt" has a list of other hidden chemicals. These chemicals include everything from manufactured forms of sodium solo-co-aluminate, iodide, sodium bicarbonate, fluoride, anticaking agents, toxic amounts of potassium iodide, and aluminum derivatives. So, the next time you go to grab that saltshaker, think of all the other little things you could be getting along with it. I'm here to shout it out to you! You don't have to rely solely on salt to get your iodine. But if you insist on "salting" your foods, go a must healthier, more natural route—Himalayan sea salt or Celtic sea salt. The benefits of getting enough iodine is that your metabolism will be able to function more properly. We are on a sodium overload with all the processed foods. Read labels. Watch your sodium intake from prepackaged foods. Try to avoid prepackaged foods. Good rule of thumb: if it came from a plant, eat it; if it was made in a plant, don't. You have plenty of food options to pick from that are naturally high in iodine. They range from seafood to potatoes, and it's nice to be able to have a variety of different foods. Even better news: everything on this list, you can eat to help your thyroid become healthier. Our bodies need an average of 150 micrograms of iodine per day.

1 medium baked organic potato with skin, 60 micrograms of iodine

Dried seaweed (1/4 ounce), 4,500 micrograms of iodine

Cod fish (3 ounces), 99 micrograms of iodine

Shrimp (3 ounces), 35 micrograms of iodine

Himalayan crystal salt (1/2 gram), 250 micrograms of iodine

Baked turkey breast (3 ounces), 34 micrograms of iodine

Dried prunes (5 prunes), 13 micrograms of iodine

Navy beans (1/2 cup), 32 micrograms of iodine

Fish sticks (2 fish sticks), 35 micrograms of iodine

Tuna in water (3 ounces), 17 micrograms of iodine

Boiled eggs (1 large egg), 12 micrograms of iodine

Plain yogurt (1 cup), 154 micrograms of iodine

Bananas (1 medium banana), 3 micrograms of iodine

Lobster (100 grams), 100 micrograms of iodine

Cheddar cheese (1 ounce), 12 micrograms of iodine

Cranberries (4 ounces), 400 micrograms of iodine

Green beans (1/2 cup), 3 micrograms of iodine

Never lose an opportunity of urging a practical beginning, however small, for it is wonderful how often in such matters the mustard-seed germinates and roots itself.

—*Florence Nightingale*

Breakfast

Breakfast is the most important meal of the day. Breakfast" literally means the meal that "breaks the fast". You've been sleeping all night fasting. Your body needs to be rebooted. You've got to "jump-start" that metabolism. Eating a healthy breakfast has been medically proven to have many health benefits, including weight control , reducing the risk of obesity , it certainly will boost your fiber intake to help you reach your daily goal of 20 to 35 grams (for adults). Eating breakfast has been shown to improve performance, have heart health advantages, helps you avoid fluctuating glucose levels, which can lead to diabetes later in life, helps you consume less calories throughout the day, so you're not binge eating of starvation at lunch time. It will give you that mental edge by enhancing your memory, your clarity, and the speed in which you are processing information, your reasoning skills, your creativity and how you absorb information. Scientists at the University of Milan in Italy reviewed 15 studies and found some evidence that those benefits. One theory suggested that if you eat a healthy breakfast it can reduce hunger throughout the day, and help you make better food choices at other meals. You should eat no later than 2 hours of waking up. Also, if you skip breakfast your hunger hormones are boosted and it can also throw your body into survival mode. Which in return starts breaking down protein in your muscles and your muscles will slowly start to break down.   Now, I hope you see the importance of why eating a healthy breakfast is so important.

Feed your family and get them out the door in a flash with these family-friendly breakfasts. Some of these you can make ahead and let the kids help you prepare it.

Banana Chocolate Overnight Oats

2 cups GF steel cut or rolled oats (steel cut for a crunch or rolled oats for a smoother oatmeal)

1 1/2 cups of almond or coconut milk

1/2 cups almond or coconut yogurt

1–2 tablespoon cocoa

1 tablespoon of ground flaxseed (omega-3 fatty acids)

1 tablespoon raw honey or grade B maple syrup Pour the mixture into two 8-ounce mason jars with lids, seal tightly, and refrigerate for at least 6 hours, preferably overnight. When ready to eat, give the oats a good shake and dig in!

Honey-Lime Fruit Salad

This easy-to-make breakfast is full of vitamins and antioxidants

2 cups chopped seasonal fruits

(I use red grapes, kiwis, mandarins, and bananas)

1 teaspoon lime juice

1 tablespoon organic honey

Combine all the ingredients in a mixing bowl.

Vegetable Quiche

1 bell pepper

2 red onions

1/2 zucchini

3 eggs

1 clove garlic, minced

Fresh parsley leaves (a handful)

3 tablespoon raw, unfiltered coconut oil

Preheat oven to 350°F. Chop vegetables and sauté in 1 1/2 tbsp. oil on medium heat for 3–4 minutes then add to a well-oiled oven-proof dish. Mix parsley, garlic and eggs in a bowl. Now pour over the vegetables and bake for 25 minutes or until firm in the center.

Mini Apple Crisp

1 medium organic apple

1 tablespoon brown sugar

1 tablespoon oats

1/2 teaspoon cinnamon

Heat oven to 350°F. Peel and core the apple and chop into 1/4-inch squares. Mix in a small bowl with sugar, oats, and cinnamon and put into a small baking dish, or line a muffin pan with paper cups. Bake for 15 minutes.

3-Ingredient Pancake Mix

1 banana

2 eggs

1 teaspoon of Ceylon cinnamon

2 tablespoons of Earth Balance butter

Mix all ingredients. Melt butter in a cast-iron skillet. Pour silver-dollar-size amounts of batter in pan. Cook 60 seconds and flip to cook the other side.

Morning Milkshake

What kid doesn't want to have a milk shake for breakfast? This is an easy and way to sneak a healthy meal!

1 cup almond milk

1 tablespoon raw honey

1 tablespoon all natural peanut butter or almond butter

1 banana, frozen (or fresh bananas and add a handful of ice cubes)

1/4 tsp. cinnamon

1 tablespoon of freshly ground flax seeds or prepared grounded flax seed mill

Combine all ingredients in a blender and blend until smooth.

Green "Thank the Goddess" Smoothie

1 cup cucumber chunks, peeled

1/2 avocado, peeled and cut into chunks

1 large kiwi, peeled and cut into chunks

1/2 cup fresh OJ

1/4 cup of fresh mint leaves

1 cup of romaine lettuce

4 pitted, dried apricots

5 ice cubes

This a delicious, easy drink to make. Add all ingredients into the blender and voila! If it's too thick, add some more freshly squeezed OJ.

Happy-Skin Smoothie

Try something different: freeze 1/2 cup of pure pumpkin (not pumpkin pie mix) in an ice cube tray.

1/2 cup of ice-cubed pure pumpkin

7 oz of So Delicious Greek-style coconut milk yogurt

1/2 cup of vita coconut water

2 tablespoons of flaxseed meal

1/2 teaspoon pumpkin spice pie mix

This a delicious, easy drink to make. Add all ingredients into the blender and voila! Your skin, thyroid, and body will thank you. And voila!

Cranberry Orange Steel Cut Oats

3 cups water

1 cup almond milk

1 tablespoon coconut oil

1 cup gluten free steel-cut oats

Sprinkle of Himalayan salt

Juice and zest from one whole orange

1/2 cup cranberries, crushed

Top with raw pumpkin seeds

Add your water and milk in a large saucepan. Simmer over medium heat. Next melt the coconut oil in a 12-inch skillet over medium heat.

Add your oats and toast, stirring occasionally, until golden and fragrant, around 1½ to 2 minutes. Stir in your oats into the simmering water/milk mixture. Reduce your heat to medium low and simmer gently for about 20 minutes, cook until the mixture is very thick. Add the salt. Continue to cook the mixture, stirring frequently, for about 10 minutes or until almost all the liquid is absorbed. Mix in the orange juice and zest. Ladle in to bowls and top with cranberries and raw pumpkin seeds.

Almond oatmeal

½ cup no sugar applesauce

2 tablespoons almond butter

2 tablespoons coconut milk

Dash of cinnamon

Dash of nutmeg

Put all ingredients in a small saucepan over med heat. Allow it to cook until done for about 10 minutes. This would be great topped with bananas and chopped Brazil nuts.

Mushroom-stuffed Omelet

I love eating breakfast for dinner. Having mushrooms, onions, and eggs are a great way to boost selenium levels. Here is a quick recipe that is both filling and super easy to whip up.

Ingredients:

4 organic or cage free eggs

3 medium-sized mushrooms, diced

½ tablespoon coconut oil or ½ tablespoon of avocado oil

A teaspoon of dairy free and soy free butter

Salt and pepper to taste

Directions:

In a cast iron skillet add a ½ tablespoon of coconut oil or avocado oil and sauté the mushrooms till they are golden brown. While mushrooms are browning.

Whisk eggs with seasonings in a bowl. After the mushrooms have browned. Add the teaspoon of butter. Stir the butter around the pan so it can get completely coated and mixed with the mushrooms.

Add the egg mixture, it will take about 1 minute for the egg to set and then flip over. Heat for another 30 seconds, then remove from pan. Place on a plate.

Overnight Pumpkin Pie Chia Pudding

2 cups coconut milk

1 cup cooked pumpkin puree

3 TBS grade B maple syrup OR raw honey

1 tsp vanilla extract

½ tsp cinnamon powder

¼ tsp ginger powder

¼ tsp allspice

4 TBS chia seeds

OPTIONAL TOPPING

Fresh fruit

Shredded coconut

Place all ingredients, except for chia seeds, into a blender and puree until smooth. Place the chia seeds into a mason jar, pour pumpkin pie flavored liquid over seeds. Seal the Mason jar with a lid and shake it good to mix well. Place in fridge the night and the next morning you will have amazing pumpkin pie pudding.

Soups and Salads

Eat salads in place of meals as much as possible. You can make your salads crispy, chewy, colorful and fun to eat. Most people enjoy eating salads--even kids! It's hard to believe that something we can't even digest can be so good for us! Eating a high-fiber diet can help lower cholesterol levels and prevent constipation. There is plenty of evidence that nutrient-rich plant foods contribute to overall health. Adding little good fat found in olive oil, avocado and nuts along with your vegetables helps your body absorb protective phytochemicals, like lycopene from tomatoes and lutein from dark green vegetables. This combination of vitamins supports the immune system, protects bones and keeps the cardiovascular system healthy.

You want to stick to homemade vinaigrettes, which are very easy to make. A great, easy-to-remember ratio is 1 part acid to 1 part oil. You don't even have to measure it if you're using a glass jar or container. Just size up an equal measure of each, then add a teaspoon or two of Dijon mustard. You can also add a dash of some salt and pepper to your taste, put on the lid, and shake. Make enough dressing to flavor your salad without drowning them in dressing. Try to experiment with different citrus juices, vinegars, flavored salts, and mustards, even a little honey. Try using your blender to make bigger batches of vinaigrette involving ingredients you'd normally have to chop like herbs, peppers, or capers. Your healthy homemade dressing will keep in the fridge for up to two weeks in a tightly sealed jar.

Chickpea Veggie Salad-in-a-Jar

This fills one 32 oz. Mason jar. Make sure to wash & dry your veggies before using.

1 oz. goat cheese

½ cup cooked, cold quinoa

1 bell pepper, chopped

1 cucumber, chopped

4 oz. grape or cherry tomatoes

5 oz. chickpeas, rinsed & dried

Dressing:

3 tsp olive oil

1 tsp white vinegar

Splash of lemon juice

Sprinkle of black pepper

Whisk dressing in a small bowl, then transfer to the bottom of the jar. Layer chickpeas on dressing. Add tomatoes, add cucumber, add bell pepper, add quinoa and top with goat cheese. Secure lid on tightly until ready to eat. Shake the salad just before eating.

Layered Quinoa Salad-in-a-Jar

This fills one 32 oz. Mason jar. Make sure to wash & dry your veggies before using.

3 Tbsp. avocado cilantro-Lime Vinaigrette

½ cup black beans, rinsed & dried

¼ cup cherry tomatoes

½ of a green pepper, chopped

½ cup cooked, cold quinoa

¼ cup organic romaine lettuce

Place the dressing in the bottom of the jar. Next add the black beans, add the tomatoes, add the peppers, add the quinoa and then add the chopped romaine. Try not to pack it in too tight, or you won't have room to shake the dressings when you are ready to eat. Seal the lid on & store in the fridge. When ready (with the lid on) shake the jar to mix everything.

Avocado Cilantro Lime Vinaigrette

½ cup extra-virgin olive oil

1 cup cilantro

¼ tsp of minced garlic

The juice of 1 orange

The juice of 3 limes

1 avocado

Salt & pepper to taste

Combine all ingredients into a blender or food processor

Puree until smooth

Mediterranean Quinoa with Seasonal Vegetables Salad-in-a-jar

This fills one 32 oz. Mason jar. You could divide this up into smaller jars. Make sure to wash & dry your veggies before using.

1 cup quinoa, rinsed well

2 cups vegetable broth

1 zucchini, diced

1 cup of corn

½ cup cherry tomatoes, diced

¼ cup red onion, diced

Vinaigrette:

2 teaspoons whole grain mustard

3 tablespoons freshly squeezed lemon juice

1 tablespoon Bragg's organic apple cider vinegar

2 garlics clove, finely minced

1/4 teaspoon crushed red pepper flakes

Freshly ground black pepper to taste

1/2 cup extra-virgin olive oil

Roast zucchini and onions, uncovered, for 20 minutes. Stir vegetables and add tomatoes and corn. Continuing roasting until tomatoes collapse, about 10 minutes. Remove vegetables and set aside

Vinaigrette

In a medium bowl whisk together mustard, lemon juice, Braggs vinegar, garlic, red pepper flakes, salt and pepper. Gradually whisk in olive oil.

Place 3 tablespoons of the dressing in the bottom of the mason jar.

Next place the roasted cooled veggies on top of the dressing and add the quinoa. Try not to pack it in too tight, or you won't have room to shake the dressings when you are ready to eat. Seal the lid on & store in the fridge. When ready (with the lid on) shake the jar to mix everything.

Roast chicken Salad-in-a-jar

This fills one 32 oz. Mason jar. Make sure to wash & dry your veggies before using.

3 Tbsp. balsamic Vinaigrette

½ cup button mushrooms, sliced

¼ cup cherry tomatoes

½ of a red onion, minced

½ cup cooked, cold roasted chicken, diced

¼ cup organic romaine lettuce

Place the dressing in the bottom of the jar. Next add the mushrooms, add the tomatoes, add the onions, add the roast chicken and then add the chopped romaine. To make it easier on me, I buy a whole, hot roasted chicken from the deli at my local grocery store. Try not to pack it in too tight, or you won't have room to shake the dressings when you are ready to eat. Seal the lid on & store in the fridge. When ready (with the lid on) shake the jar to mix everything.

Balsamic Vinaigrette

3 tablespoons balsamic vinegar

1 tablespoon Dijon mustard

1 garlic clove, minced

1/2 cup olive oil

Salt and freshly ground pepper

In a small bowl, combine the vinegar, mustard, and garlic. Add the oil in a slow steady stream, whisking constantly. Season with salt and pepper to taste.

Layered Taco Salad-in-a-jar

This fills one 32 oz. Mason jar. Make sure to wash & dry your veggies before using.

¼ cup cucumber, diced

1 roma tomato, diced

½ cup black beans, rinsed and drained

¼ cup corn

¼ red bell pepper, diced

¼ cup avocado, diced

1 cup of romaine lettuce, chopped

2 tablespoon of goat cheese

Cilantro-lime dressing

1 tablespoon apple cider vinegar

Juice from 1 lime

½ cup fresh cilantro

¼ cup nonfat Greek yogurt (I have a recipe for nondairy yogurt in the back) 1 teaspoon raw honey

Blend the salad dressing until smooth and pour it in the bottom of your mason jar. Next layer you salad from heaviest to lightest. Add your cucumbers, then your tomatoes, next your black beans and your corn. On top of that place your red bell pepper, next your avocado. Lastly place your lettuce and then the cheese on top of that. Try not to pack it in too tight, or you won't have room to shake the dressings when you are ready to eat. Seal the lid on & store in the fridge. When ready (with the lid on) shake the jar to mix everything.

Grilled Chicken, Beet, Apple Salad-in –a-jar

This fills one 32 oz. Mason jar. Make sure to wash & dry your veggies before using.

1 beets, scrubbed, peeled and diced into small bite size pieces

1 teaspoon olive oil

Salt and pepper to taste

¼ cup roasted chicken breast, diced

1/2 apple, washed and diced

2 cups organic romaine lettuce

1 ounce goat cheese

¼ cup raw pumpkin seeds

Strawberry Vinaigrette

1/4 cup fresh strawberries

1/2 tablespoon olive oil

1/2 tablespoon balsamic vinegar

Pinch of salt

Pinch of ground black pepper

1/4 teaspoon raw honey

Blend the salad dressing until smooth and pour it in the bottom of your mason jar. Next layer you salad from heaviest to lightest. Add your beets, then your chicken and your diced apples. Lastly place your lettuce, next the goat cheese, then your raw pumpkin seeds. Try not to pack it in too tight, or you won't have room to shake the dressings when you are ready to eat. Seal the lid on & store in the fridge. When ready (with the lid on) shake the jar to mix everything.

Smoked Salmon Salad-a-Jar

This fills one 32 oz. Mason jar. Make sure to wash & dry your veggies before using.

¼ cup smoked salmon, diced

¼ cup cucumbers, diced

2 carrots shredded

¼ cup red onion, diced

2 cups organic romaine lettuce

Lemony vinaigrette

3 tablespoons olive oil

1 tablespoon white balsamic vinegar

1/2 Meyer lemon, zested and juiced

In a small bowl, whisk together olive oil, vinegar, lemon juice, and of lemon juice with the zest. Pour in the bottom of your mason jar.

Next add the cucumbers, carrots, red onion, salmon and lettuce. Try not to pack it in too tight, or you won't have room to shake the dressings when you are ready to eat. Seal the lid on & store in the fridge. When ready (with the lid on) shake the jar to mix everything.

Spring Artichoke Salad

1/4 pound red potatoes, quartered

1/2 pound green beans, cut into 2-inch pieces

2- 6 oz. jars marinated artichoke quarters (keep 2 Tablespoons of the marinade)

3 Tablespoons olive oil

2 Tablespoons fresh lemon juice

1 teaspoon Dijon mustard

2 Tablespoons parsley, chopped

2 teaspoons dried oregano

2 teaspoons orange zest

1 cup cherry tomatoes, halved

Salt, to taste

Pepper, to taste

Blanch your green beans in a boiling water green beans until crisp and tender, about 1 minute. Remove the beans from the hot water with a slotted spoon and place in a bowl of cold water. After you've removed the beans add your diced red potatoes to the same water and allow them to cook until they are tender. Next, remove the beans from the cold water after a minute this stops the cooking process and pat the beans dry to remove excess water. Once the potatoes have cooked for about 8 minutes, remove them from the water and drain. Drain the liquid out of the artichoke hearts, reserving 2 Tablespoons of the marinade. In a bowl, add the reserved 2 Tablespoons of artichoke marinade, plus the olive oil, lemon juice, Dijon mustard, parsley and oregano. Whisk together until combined. Next add the potatoes, green beans, artichoke hearts and cherry tomatoes to the bowl of dressing and toss to combine well. Season with your Himalayan sea salt or Celtic sea salt and pepper to taste. Serve chilled or at room temperature.

Quinoa Chickpea and Avocado Salad

1 cup quartered grape tomatoes

15-ounce can garbanzo beans, rinsed and drained

1 cup cooked quinoa

2 tablespoon red onion, minced

2 tablespoon cilantro, minced

1 1/2 limes, juiced

Himalayan sea salt or Celtic sea salt

1 cup diced cucumber

4 oz. diced avocado (1 medium Hass)

Combine all the ingredients except for avocado and cucumber. Next season with salt and pepper to taste. Keep refrigerated until ready to serve. Just Before serving, add cucumber and avocado.

Smoked Turkey Salad-in-a-Jar

This fills one 32 oz. Mason jar. Make sure to wash & dry your veggies before using.

3 tablespoons of raspberry balsamic vinaigrette

¼ cup smoked turkey, diced

¼ cup cucumbers, diced

¼ cup cherry tomatoes, diced

2 boiled eggs, diced

5 tbsp. Walnuts, raw

2 cups organic romaine lettuce

Raspberry Vinaigrette Dressing

1 cup of fresh raspberries

¼ cup olive oil

2/3 cup balsamic vinegar

1 tablespoon of honey

Blend everything until smooth.

Pour 3 tablespoons of the vinaigrette in the bottom of your mason jar. Next add your cucumbers, cherry tomatoes, turkey, romaine lettuce, boiled eggs and walnuts. Try not to pack it in too tight, or you won't have room to shake the dressings when you are ready to eat. Seal the lid on & store in the fridge. When ready (with the lid on) shake the jar to mix everything

Cajun Shrimp salad-in-a-jar

¼ cup sautéed bell peppers, diced

¼ cup sautéed onions, diced

¼ cup Cajun shrimp, cooked

¼ cup freshly smashed guacamole

½ cup Boston Bibb lettuce

Sautee your bell peppers and onions in extra virgin olive oil. Set aside. Next sauté your shrimp in dash of paprika, garlic granules, chili powder, cayenne, and Himalayan sea salt. Cook until completely pink. You want to buy shrimp that is already deveined and the tails are cut off.

Sweet Potato Soup

2lbs of sweet potatoes, chopped

1 onion, diced

1 carrot, diced

1 tsp of minced garlic

3 cups of chicken stock

½ cup coconut milk

Place everything in a slow cooker except for the coconut milk. Cook on low for 6 or high for 4. Puree smooth then add the coconut milk and cook an additional 30 minutes.

Slow Cooker Quinoa, Chicken and Butternut Squash Soup

1 medium butternut squash, peeled and cubed

14 oz. can coconut milk, full fat

2 cups water

2 tbsp. raw honey or maple syrup

1 tbsp. red curry paste

1 inch ginger, peeled & grated

1 garlic clove, crushed

1 1/2 tsp salt

1.5 lbs. chicken breast

2 cups quinoa, cooked

2 large red bell peppers, thinly sliced

1/4 cup cilantro, chopped

1/2 lime, juice of

In a large slow cooker, add squash, coconut milk, water, honey, curry paste, ginger, garlic, salt, lime leaves and chicken. Cover and cook on Low for 8 hours or on High for 4 hours. Remove chicken and shred using two forks. Using immersion blender, blend soup until smooth. Add chicken, quinoa, bell peppers, cilantro and lime juice. Stir and enjoy!

"Creamy" Chicken Tomato Soup Slow Cooker

4 frozen skinless boneless chicken breast

Garlic salt to taste

2 tablespoons Italian Seasoning

1 tablespoon dried basil

1 clove garlic

1 14 oz. can of coconut milk (full fat)

1 14 oz. can diced tomatoes and juice

1 cup of chicken broth

Sea Salt and pepper to taste

Put all the above ingredients into the crock-pot, cook for 9 hours on low. After 9 hours take two forks and shred the chicken, set the crock-pot on warm till ready to serve. For a creamier soup, before adding back the shredded chicken. Blend some of the soup and put it back in the slow cooker. You can this in batches in a regular blend but remember it's hot or use an immersion hand held blender.

Dinner Dishes

Spaghetti Squash & Turkey Meatballs

1 3-pound spaghetti squash

2 tablespoons water

2 tablespoons extra-virgin olive oil, divided

1/2 cup chopped fresh parsley, divided

1 1/4 teaspoons Italian seasoning, divided

1/2 teaspoon onion powder

1/2 teaspoon salt, divided

1/2 teaspoon freshly ground pepper

1 pound 93%-lean ground turkey

4 large cloves garlic, minced

1 28-ounce can no-salt-added crushed tomatoes

1/4-1/2 teaspoon crushed red pepper

Halve squash lengthwise and scoop out the seeds. Place face down in a microwave-safe dish; add ¼ cup water. Microwave, uncovered, on High until the flesh can be easily scraped with a fork, 10 to 15 minutes.

Heat 1 tablespoon oil in a large skillet over medium-high heat. Scrape the squash flesh into the skillet and cook, stirring occasionally, until the moisture is evaporated and the squash is beginning to brown, 5 to 10 minutes. Stir in 1/4 cup parsley. Remove from heat, cover and let stand.

Meanwhile, combine the remaining 1/4 cup parsley, 1/2 teaspoon Italian seasoning, onion powder, 1/4 teaspoon salt and pepper in a medium bowl. Add turkey; gently mix to combine (do not overmix). Using about 2 tablespoons each, form into 12 meatballs.

Heat the remaining 1 tablespoon oil in a large nonstick skillet over medium-high heat. Add the meatballs, reduce heat to medium and cook, turning occasionally, until browned all over, 4 to 6 minutes. Push the meatballs to the side of the pan, add garlic and cook, stirring, for 1 minute. Add tomatoes, crushed red pepper to taste, the remaining 3/4 teaspoon Italian seasoning and 1/4 teaspoon salt; stir to coat the meatballs. Bring to a simmer, cover and cook, stirring occasionally, until the meatballs are cooked through, 10 to 12 minutes more.

Serve the sauce and meatballs over the squash.

Garlic Shrimp with Cilantro Spaghetti Squash

1 2 1/2- to 3-pound spaghetti squash, halved lengthwise and seeded

2 tablespoons extra-virgin olive oil

1 tablespoon minced garlic

- 1 teaspoon ground coriander
- 1 teaspoon ground cumin
- 1/2 teaspoon salt, divided
- 1/4 teaspoon cayenne pepper
- 1/3 cup dry white wine
- 1 pound peeled and deveined raw shrimp (16-20 per pound), tails left on if desired
- 1 tablespoon lemon juice
- 1/4 cup chopped fresh cilantro
- 2 tablespoons non-dairy butter, melted
- 1/4 teaspoon ground pepper
- Lemon wedges for serving

Halve squash lengthwise and scoop out the seeds. Place face down in a microwave-safe dish; add ¼ cup water. Microwave, uncovered, on High until the flesh can be easily scraped with a fork, 10 to 15 minutes. Next heat oil in a large skillet over medium-high heat. Add garlic, coriander, cumin, 1/4 teaspoon salt and cayenne; cook, stirring, for 30 seconds. Add wine and bring to a simmer. Add shrimp and cook, stirring, until the shrimp are pink and just cooked through, 3 to 4 minutes. Remove from heat and stir in lemon juice.

Use a fork to scrape the squash from the shells into a medium bowl. Add cilantro, butter, pepper and the remaining 1/4 teaspoon salt; stir to combine. Serve the shrimp over the spaghetti squash with a lemon wedge on the side.

Oven-Fried Salmon Cakes over a bed of Quinoa Pilaf

1 (14.75 ounce) can wild-caught pink or red salmon

1 cup cooked (or canned) sweet potato, mashed

2 large eggs, beaten

1/2 cup almond flour

1/2 cup fresh parsley leaves, minced (about 2 tablespoons)

2 scallions, white and green, very thinly sliced

1 tablespoon Old Bay Seasoning

1 teaspoon salt

1 teaspoon hot sauce

1/2 teaspoon paprika

1/4 teaspoon ground black pepper

Zest from 1 lemon

2 tablespoons non-dairy butter, melted

Preheat the oven to 425F and cover a large baking sheet with parchment paper. Drain the liquid from the salmon and using your fingers, crumble the fish into a large mixing bowl, removing the bones and flaking the fish. Add the sweet potato, eggs, almond flour, parsley, scallions, Old Bay Seasoning, salt, hot pepper sauce, paprika, black pepper, and lemon zest. Mix well and refrigerate for 10 minutes.

Brush the parchment paper with some of the melted non-dairy butter, then use a 1/3 measuring cup to scoop the cakes and drop them onto the parchment. The patties should be about 2 1/2 inches wide and about 1 inch thick. Brush the tops of the cakes with the nondairy butter, then bake for 20 minutes. Carefully flip each patty with a spatula and return to the oven. Bake an additional 10 minutes until golden brown and crisp. Serve with a squeeze of lemon juice and your sauce of choice.

Baked chicken and sweet potato casserole

1lb of chicken, cubed and diced

2 teaspoon of mustard

3tablepoons of evvo

2 medium sweet potatoes, peeled and diced

Salt & pepper to season

Preheat oven to 425. Diced your chicken into cubes and mix the diced chicken in a bowl with mustard and evoo. Sautee your diced chicken in a pan until it is no longer pink on the outside. Place your precooked chicken in a baking dish. Mix your diced sweet potatoes with your chicken. Season with salt n pepper and cook for 25 minutes until sweet potatoes are tender & chicken is cooked through.

Artichoke Rosemary Chicken

4 lb boneless, skinless chicken breast (trimmed of any extra tendons or fat) and cut into thirds

4 fresh artichoke hearts (halved) or 2 cups of canned artichoke hearts

1 medium red onion, sliced

1 lb. baby portabella mushrooms, halved or quartered

4 Tbsp. horseradish mustard or brown mustard

6-8 cloves fresh garlic, minced

1/4 cup extra virgin olive oil

1/2 cup balsamic vinegar

1/2 cup white wine

1 teaspoon dried basil

1/2 teaspoon dried thyme

1 teaspoon dried rosemary

Himalayan sea salt and black pepper to taste

Place your cut up chicken in a large glass casserole baking pan. Evenly place the artichoke hearts, onions, and mushrooms. Sprinkle to taste with pepper and salt.

In a small bowl mix together the mustard, garlic, olive oil, balsamic vinegar, white wine, basil, thyme, and rosemary. Pour the liquid over the chicken/artichoke/onions. Bake at 350 degrees for 75 minutes. Serve with brown rice or rosemary sweet potatoes.

One pot Skillet chili mac n cheese

1 tablespoon olive oil

2 cloves garlic, minced

1 onion diced

1 red bell pepper, diced

1 lb. of grass fed beef

4 cups of low sodium chicken broth

1 (14.5) toasted diced tomatoes

1 can of white kidney beans, rinsed well

1 can of red kidney beans, rinsed well

3 teaspoons of chili powder

10 ounces of uncooked elbow brown rice pasta

¾ cup of goats cheese

Place your EVOO in a large skillet or Dutch oven over medium heat. Add garlic, onion and ground beef, and cook until browned, about 3-5 minutes, making sure to crumble the beef as it cooks; drain excess fat. Next pour in chicken broth, tomatoes, beans, chili powder and cumin; season with salt n pepper. Bring to a simmer & stir in pasta. Reduce heat and cover allow to simmer for 15 minutes until pasta is tender.

One Pan Ranch Pork Chops and Veggies

4 (8-ounce) pork chops, bone-in, 3/4-inch to 1-inch thick

16 ounces baby red potatoes, halved

16 ounces green beans, trimmed

2 tablespoons olive oil

1 (1-ounce) package Ranch Seasoning and Salad Dressing Mix

3 cloves garlic, minced

Himalayan sea salt and freshly ground black pepper, to taste

2 tablespoons chopped fresh parsley leaves

Preheat oven to 400 degrees F. Lightly oil a baking pan.

Place pork chops, potatoes and green beans in a single layer onto the prepared baking pan. Drizzle with olive oil and sprinkle with Ranch Seasoning and garlic; season with salt and pepper, to taste.

Place into oven and roast until the pork is completely cooked through, reaching an internal temperature of 140 degrees F, about 20-22 minutes. Next turn on the broiler and broil for 2-3 minutes, or until caramelized and slightly charred.

Garlic Zucchini Noodles w/ meat balls

2 zucchinis, cleaned

1 tablespoon EVOO

¼ teaspoon garlic powder

¼ teaspoon garlic salt

1 pound lean ground chicken, turkey or beef

4 large cloves garlic, minced

1 28-ounce can no-salt-added crushed tomatoes

1/4-1/2 teaspoon crushed red pepper

Pepper to taste

Spiralize your zucchini.

Meanwhile, combine the remaining 1/4 cup parsley, 1/2 teaspoon Italian seasoning, onion powder, 1/4 teaspoon salt and pepper in a medium bowl. Add ground chicken. ; Gently mix to combine (do not overmix). Using about 2 tablespoons each, form into 12 meatballs.

Heat the remaining 1 tablespoon oil in a large nonstick skillet over medium-high heat. Add the meatballs, reduce heat to medium and cook, turning occasionally, until browned all over, 4 to 6 minutes. Push the meatballs to the side of the pan, add garlic and cook, stirring, for 1 minute. Add tomatoes, crushed red pepper to taste, the remaining 3/4 teaspoon Italian seasoning and 1/4 teaspoon salt; stir to coat the meatballs. Bring to a simmer, cover and cook, stirring occasionally, until the meatballs are cooked through, 10 to 12 minutes more.

In another skillet on the stove over medium heat.

Once pan is hot, add EVOO and zoodles. Let sauté for about a minute, then add in the seasonings. Cook additional 2-3 minutes. Zoodles should be soft, but still have a slight stiffness. Next incorporate the zoodles and the meatball/sauce mixture and gentle mix.

Oven Baked Fajita

1 pound boneless, skinless chicken breasts, cut into strips

2 Tbsp. coconut oil, melted

2 tsp chili powder

1 1/2 tsp cumin

1/2 tsp garlic powder

1/2 tsp dried oregano

1/4 tsp seasoned salt

1 (15 oz) can diced tomatoes with green chilies

1 medium onion, sliced

1/2 red bell pepper, cut into strips

1/2 green bell pepper, cut into strips

Place chicken strips in a greased 13×9 baking dish. Preheat your oven to 400 degrees.

In a bowl mix the oil, chili powder, cumin, garlic powder, dried oregano, and salt.

Mix the seasoning over the chicken and stir to coat.

Next add the tomatoes, peppers, and onions to the dish and stir to combine.

Bake uncovered for 20-25 minutes or until chicken is cooked through and the vegetables are tender. You can eat this in a large lettuce leaf.

Snacks

Coconut Flour Cupcakes

½ cup melted coconut oil

⅔ Cup coconut sugar

½ teaspoon Himalayan salt

2 teaspoons vanilla extract

6 large eggs

2 Tablespoons water

½ cup coconut flour

1 teaspoon baking powder

Preheat your oven to 350º. Whisk oil sugar, salt, vanilla, eggs, and water. Next add in the coconut flour and baking powder. Add your egg mixture in with the flour mixture and make sure its combined well. Place a dozen paper cupcake in your muffin pan. Fill each cup ¾ full.

Bake your cupcakes on the center rack of the oven for 18-20 minutes, until a toothpick inserted into the center of a cupcake comes out clean. After you remove the cupcakes from oven allow them to cool for 5 minutes. Make sure you allow them to cool completely before you add your icing.

Banana-Coconut Raw Vegan Ice Cream

6 bananas, frozen and cut into pieces

½ cup shredded coconut

¼ teaspoon 100% Pure Vanilla Powder

Place your bananas in a high speed blender. I have a Vitamix but a food processor will work too. Blend until they're smooth and creamy. Don't blend for too long or the ice cream will begin to melt. Next add the shredded coconut and vanilla and blend for 30 seconds or until the coconut and vanilla are thoroughly mixed into the ice cream. Serve in bowls and you can add melted chocolate or other toppings on top!

Dark Chocolate coconut apricot bites

5 dried Apricots

1/2 ounce dark chocolate

Sprinkle some coarse Celtic sea salt and shredded coconut

Lay a piece of parchment paper on a plate. Heat dark chocolate in a small bowl in the microwave at 20 second intervals. Stir often and heat until JUST melted (chocolate burns easily in the microwave). Dip 1/2 apricot in the chocolate, put on plate, and dust with salt. Refrigerate for 1/2 hour and serve.

No-bake oatmeal bites

 1 cup dry quick oats

2/3 cup coconut flakes

1/2 cup almond butter

1/2 cup dark chocolate chips

1/3 cup raw honey

1 tsp vanilla

Directions: Mix all ingredients, form into 1 inch balls. Place balls in refrigerator and snack away.

Fried Chickpeas

2 teaspoons smoked paprika

1 teaspoon cayenne pepper

6 tablespoons extra-virgin olive oil

2 15-oz. cans chickpeas, rinsed, drained, patted very dry

Kosher salt

2 teaspoons finely grated lime zest

Combine paprika and cayenne in a small bowl and set aside.

Heat oil in a cast iron skillet over medium-high heat. Working in 2 batches, add chickpeas to skillet and sauté, stirring frequently, until golden and crispy, 15–20 minutes. Using a slotted spoon, transfer chickpeas to paper towels to get excess oil off. Transfer to a bowl. Sprinkle paprika mixture over; toss to coat. Season to taste with salt. Toss with lime zest and serve. You can eat this over a bowl of brown rice or quinoa.

Spicy pumpkin seeds

Dash of Himalayan sea salt

1 teaspoon of coconut oil

¼ teaspoon of smoked paprika

¼ teaspoon of garlic powder

1/8 teaspoon of chili powder

1 cup of raw pumpkin seeds

Melt coconut oil. Mix everything with the seeds in a bowl. Lay seeds on a baking dish. Roast for 20 minutes tossing after 10. Make sure they don't become overly brown. That means the inside of the seed is burning.

Salad Dressings

Many over-the-counter condiments, sauces and salad dressings are filled with Trans fats, sugar, preservatives, and artificial ingredients and flavors. You will be amazed if you started to read labels. You would see words like calcium disodium EDTA, canola oil (and/or soybean oil), caramel color, cellulose gum, cornstarch (or modified cornstarch), disodium guanylate, disodium inosinate, gum arabic, MSG (monosodium glutamate), polysorbate 60, potassium sorbate, sodium and calcium caseinates. Making your own condiments, sauces and salad dressings is easy. All it takes is a little extra time. Do you want your condiments, sauces or salad dressing to come from a lab or your kitchen? All the recipes can be prepared ahead and refrigerated in a mason jar with a tightly sealed lid up to 1 week. You can find more of these mouthwatering recipes in my book A Survivors Guide to kicking Hypothyroidism Booty.

Red Wine Vinaigrette

2 tablespoons red wine vinegar

1 teaspoon Dijon mustard (optional)

1 small garlic clove, minced (optional)

1/3 cup extra-virgin olive oil

Coarse salt and ground pepper

Pour all the ingredients in a mason jar with a lid and give a good shake to combine. You can season with Himalayan sea salt and freshly ground black pepper. Store in refrigerator

Honey-Balsamic Vinaigrette

2 tablespoons balsamic vinegar

1 tablespoon raw honey

1 teaspoon Dijon mustard

1/4 cup extra-virgin olive oil

1 garlic glove, minced

Freshly ground black pepper and Himalayan Sea salt to taste. Pour all the ingredients in a mason jar with a lid and give a good shake to combine. You can season with Himalayan sea salt and freshly ground black pepper. Store in refrigerator.

Basic Vinaigrette

1 cup olive oil

1/4 cup organic apple cider vinegar

1 teaspoon garlic powder

1 teaspoon onion powder

1 teaspoon Celtic sea salt

1/2 teaspoon black pepper

Pour all the ingredients in a mason jar with a lid and give a good shake to combine. You can season with Himalayan sea salt and freshly ground black pepper. Store in refrigerator.

Cucumber–Coconut Milk Ranch Dressing

1 can full-fat coconut milk or coconut cream,

Refrigerated overnight

1 medium cucumber, peeled, halved lengthwise, seeded, and

Grated on the large holes of a box grater

2 tablespoons minced shallots

1 garlic clove, minced

2 tablespoons organic apple cider vinegar

3 tablespoons chopped fresh chives

1 1/2 tablespoons chopped fresh parsley

1 1/2 tablespoons chopped fresh basil

1 tablespoon chopped fresh dill

Pinch of cayenne pepper

Place a can of full-fat coconut milk in the fridge overnight this will help the cull-fat of the coconut milk go to the store and be easy to scoop out. After you've done this scoop cream off the top of the can and add it to a large mason jar. Save 4 tablespoons of the coconut water in the can and add it to the hard coconut cream and mix together until smooth. Don't discard the other coconut water. If the mixture is thick you always add more coconut to thin it out. Add the remaining ingredients to your mason jar. Close lid tightly, shake until combined and refrigerate dressing for at least 30 minutes to let the flavors combine together. Keep in the refrigerator after you use it to remain fresh.

Tell me what you eat, and I will tell you what you are.

— Anthelme Brillat-Savarin (1755–1826)

The Physiology of Taste

Final words and thoughts from the Author:

Changing your habits to become a better you.

One of the most inspiring facts about life is that it flows from the inside out. We're affected by what happens inside—our feelings and our thoughts— our health and our happiness all of these things play a very important role in how see view the world every day. This has a direct impact on our well-being, it can change our mindset, the words we convey, and our response with the world.

The shocking truth is YOU have the power.

I've been battling hypothyroidism for years. After many unsuccessful doctors' appointments over the years, it seemed none offered me ideas on diet change. It was here take this pill. I decided that I had to take charge of my health. You have to heal your body from the inside out. It's not about being skinny, it's about gaining energy, vitality, and feeling good when you look in the mirror. You have the power for change in your life.

You're worth it.

Sometimes your life just needs clarity. You have to step out of your comfort zone and focus on what your heart desires. If you desire to be healthier, happier or have a more fulfilled life then you need to take the steps necessary to achieve those goals. No one is going to do this better than you. No one will do this for you. You were born with the capacity of abundance. You have to clear away any of the emotional, mental, and energetic debris that is in the way of your ability to see who you really are and create the life you really deserve. Right now, you are making different choices. You deserve to this! The journey has just begun. Congratulations. You've taken your 1st steps into becoming a more beautiful you. I challenge you to find your inner strength. Focus on that vision and get a clear picture of what you want. Speak words of inspiration to your soul. Say things like, "I will do things to make a difference in my health", "I am beautiful", "I am happy". I am not going to sugar coat this it does take some work. You're unstoppable. Life is the ultimate adventure. Every day we are fill the opportunities to make an impact and have a ripple effect on our health and others around us. Be the Spark! I thank you for being curious and seeking after the truth. All of us, who were told it was all in our head, all of us who wouldn't take no for the answer and demanded a change. No more being stuck in limbo and feeling like you can't get out of this rut. You will make a difference not only in your health but the health and well-being of others. You have the power and you have the mindset.

3 things that you can do to shift your mindset. When you feel bombarded with life and things are not going your way. Stop, take a deep breathe, and write down on a piece of paper. Yes, I am going old school. Pen and paper.

1. What do you have that makes you grateful?
2. What do you love and why?

Don't just list what you love and are grateful for. List why. Embellish them. Bask in them. Be specific why you appreciate it.

3. be grateful for the small mercies in life.

Only when you open your eyes with gratitude you can honestly see the world for what it is. It is a beautiful thing!

If you compare your elf to others, please, stop that revolving door of comparison and negativity. Surround yourself with people who don't value YOU, on your looks but your heart and self-worth.

Become SOUL FOOD!

Be someone who brings value to other's lives. Someone who lifts others up when they are down. Someone who doesn't judge. Someone who looks for beauty beyond skin deep.

Which do you think would make you feel happy, valuable, and whole?

We have been programmed since birth by the world around us on how we look. Especially as women, we play the "comparison" game with all the celebrity and supermodel bodies while we are swamped with in social media, t.v. programs and movies.

I am guilty of playing the "comparison" game with how I looked, and I have been in situations in the past that truly made me feel like I was "eye candy." My heart didn't matter, MY goals didn't matter, and MY opinion didn't matter.

So what happened to me while I was obsessed and worried about how I look? Stress, Sadness, Self-sabotage… All bad things..

Beauty radiates from the inside –out.

Become SOUL FOOD!

> If you always do what you always did, you will always get what you always got.
>
> – Albert Einstein

Let's go over some important things. We are one of the richest country in the world and we have an abundance of food everywhere it seems but yet we are extremely malnourished and mineral deficient. Why is that? We are literally starving our bodies to death. How can this be? Our problem is that even with all of this abundance of food , readily available at our hands, people aren't obtaining the basic nutrients their bodies needs in order to fuel what is needed to perform the necessary basic functions. The Standard American diet in a nutshell of unhealthy saturated fats and Trans fats, our meals are unbalanced, oversized, and loaded with cholesterol, salt, sugar, artificial ingredients and preservatives. You have to start addressing what the root cause is of your hypothyroidism. Would you take Motrin if you got a rock stuck in your shoe? Hypothyroidism does has a root issue. We often ignore the underlying cause of hypothyroidism. Sometimes we have to do a little pruning of the branches, in order for the tree to be healthy again. A number of things can be the reason why you have hypothyroidism. It could be a wide range of things from celiac disease, Hashimoto's, leaky gut, autoimmune disease disorder, nutrient deficiency's, adrenal fatigue, exposure to chemicals, gluten or other food allergies, and hormonal imbalance. It starts with the foods we eat to the chemicals in the environment, your thyroid can be influenced by many different circumstances.

 Most of your "conditions" and labels are a lack of the proper nutrition and/or vitamins and minerals. Why not do a little research and find what is causing your disorder? Look up what nutritional steps you need to start taking. What environmental things have an effect on your disorder and start avoiding that. Why not give your body a fighting chance to heal the issue at hand with herbs, specific vitamins & other natural supplements. In each stage of our lives our bodies change and we must learn to adapt and adjust what it needs. Trust me when I say, there certainly isn't a substitute for figuring out the real underlying reason for your "condition". I am not saying try this solely on your on I would recommend that you get qualified practitioner that will be able to order the appropriate tests for you, and also help you interpret them. You can click on this link and just place in your zip code. It will help you find a Naturopath Doctor in your area.

Looking at the big picture. Like an onion, you must start to work on each layer and see what needs to be addressed, peeling it back, layer by layer.

Just think how great it's going to feel when you are as healthy on the inside as you look on the outside! The ultimate goal isn't to look fit but to be fit.

I want to thank you for reading my latest book. I hope that it has enhanced and enlightened your life.

Disclaimer

The information and recipes contained in book is based upon the research and the personal experiences of the author. It's for entertainment purposes only. Every attempt has been made to provide accurate, up to date and reliable information. No warranties of any kind are expressed or implied. Readers acknowledge that the author is not engaging in the rendering of legal, financial, medical or professional advice. By reading this blog, the reader agrees that under no circumstance the author is not responsible for any loss, direct or indirect, which are incurred by using this information contained within this blog. Including but not limited to errors, omissions or inaccuracies. This blog is not intended as replacements from what your health care provider has suggested. The author is not responsible for any adverse effects or consequences resulting from the use of any of the suggestions, preparations or procedures discussed in this blog. All matters pertaining to your health should be supervised by a health care professional. I am not a doctor, or a medical professional. This blog is designed for as an educational and entertainment tool only. Please always check with your health practitioner before taking any vitamins, supplements, or herbs, as they may have side-effects, especially when combined with medications, alcohol, or other vitamins or supplements. Knowledge is power, educate yourself and find the answer to your health care needs. Wisdom is a wonderful thing to seek. I hope this blog will teach and encourage you to take leaps in your life to educate yourself for a happier & healthier life. You have to take ownership of your health.

References:

http://www.ewg.org/research/dirty-dozen-list-endocrine-disruptors

ATSDR (Agency for Toxic Substances and Disease Registry). 2004. Toxicological profile for polybrominated biphenyls and polybrominated diphenyl ethers. http://www.atsdr.cdc.gov/toxprofiles/tp.asp?id=529&tid=94

ATSDR (Agency for Toxic Substances and Disease Registry). 2009. Public Health Statement for Perfluoroalkyls. Agency for Toxic Substances and Disease Registry, Division of Toxicology and Environmental Medicine. May 2009. http://www.atsdr.cdc.gov/toxprofiles/tp200-c1-b.pdf

Blount BC, Pirkle JL, Oserloh JD, Valentin-Blasini L, Caldwell KL. 2006. Urinary perchlorate and thyroid hormone levels in adolescent and adult men and women living in the Unites States. Environmental Health Perspectives 114(12): 1865-71.

Buck Louis GM, Sundaram R, Schisterman EF, Sweeney AM, Lynch CD, Gore-Langton RE et al. 2012. Heavy metals and couple fecundity, the life study. Chemisphere 87(11): 1201-7.

Corpas I, Castillo M, Marquina D, Benito MJ. 2002. Lead intoxication in gestational and lactation periods alters the development of male reproductive organs. Ecotoxicology and Environmental Safety 53(2): 259-66.

De Coster S, van Larebeke N. 2012. Endocrine-disrupting chemicals: associated disorders and mechanisms of action. Journal of Environmental and Public Health Article ID 713696. http://www.hindawi.com/journals/jeph/2012/713696/cta/

Department of Health and Human Services, Public Health Service. September 2004. http://www.atsdr.cdc.gov/toxprofiles/tp.asp?id=529&tid=94

Dearth RK, Hiney JK, Srivastava V, Burdick SB, Bratton GR, Dees WL. 2002. Effects of lead (Pb) exposure during gestation and lactation on female pubertal development in the rat. Reproductive Toxicology 16(4): 343-52.

Du G, Hu J, Huang H, Qin Y, Han X, Wu D, et al. 2013. Perfluorooctane sulfonate (PFOS) affects hormone receptor activity, steroidogenesis, and expression of endocrine-related genes in vitro and in vivo. Environmental Toxicology and Chemistry 32(2): 353-60.

EPA (U.S. Environmental Protection Agency). 2010. Consumer Factsheet on: Dioxin. U.S. Environmental Protection Agency. August 2010. http://cfpub.epa.gov/ncea/CFM/nceaQFind.cfm?keyword=Dioxin

EPA (U.S. Environmental Protection Agency). 2012. Emerging Contaminants Fact Sheet – Perfluorooctane Sulfonate (PFOS) and Perfluorooctanoic Acid (PFOA). U.S. Environmental Protection Agency. May 2012. http://www.epa.gov/fedfac/pdf/emerging_contaminants_pfos_pfoa.pdf

EPA (U.S. Environmental Protection Agency). 2013. Consumer Factsheet on: Atrazine. U.S. Environmental Protection Agency. January 2013. http://www.epa.gov/oppsrrd1/reregistration/atrazine/atrazine_update.htm

EPA (U.S. Environmental Protection Agency). 2013. Consumer fact sheet on: GLYCOL ETHERS. U.S. Environmental Protection Agency. October 2013. http://www.epa.gov/ttnatw01/hlthef/glycolet.html

EWG (Environmental Working Group). 2003. Suspect Salads. Toxic Rocket Fuel Fond in Samples of Winter Lettuce. http://www.ewg.org/research/suspect-salads

EWG (Environmental Working Group). 2003. PFCs: Global Contaminants.

http://www.ewg.org/research/pfcs-global-contaminants

EWG (Environmental Working Group). 2004. Rocket Fuel Contamination in California Milk. http://www.ewg.org/research/rocket-fuel-cows-milk-perchlorate

Fan W, Yanase T, Morinaga H, Gondo S, Okabe T, Nomura M, et al. 2007. Atrazine-induced aromatase expression is SF-1 dependent: implications for endocrine disruption in wildlife and reproductive cancers in humans. Environmental Health Perspectives 115(5): 720-727.

FDA (Food and Drug Administration). 2013. Survey Data on Perchlorate in Food - 2005/2006 Total Diet Study Results.

http://www.fda.gov/Food/FoodborneIllnessContaminants/ChemicalContaminant...

Giammona CJ, Sawhney P, Chandrasekaran Y, Richburg JH. 2002. Death receptor response in rodent testis after mono-(2-ethylhexyl) phthalate exposure. Toxicology and Applied Pharmacology 185(2): 119-27.

http://www.healthline.com/health/t4-test

Gilbert ME, Rovet J, Chen Z, Koibuchi N. 2012. Developmental thyroid hormone disruption: prevalence, environmental contaminants and neurodevelopmental consequences. Neurotoxicology 33(4): 842-52.

Griswold MD. 1988. Protein secretions of sertoli cells. International Review of Cytology 110: 133-56.

Hardin BD, Goad PT, Burg JR. 1986. Developmental toxicity of diethylene glycol monomethyl ether (diEGME). Fundamental and Applied Toxicology: Official Journal of the Society of Toxicology 6(3):430-9.

Hayes TB, Stuart AA, Mendoza M, Collins A, Noriega N, Vonk A. 2006. Characterization of atrazine-induced gonadal malformations in african clawed frogs (Xenopus laevis) and comparisons with effects of an androgen antagonist (cyproterone acetate) and exogenous estrogen (17β estradiol): support for the demasculinization/feminization hypothesis. Environmental Health Perspectives 114(Suppl 1): 134-141.

Hayes TB, Khoury V, Narayan A, Nazir M, Park A, Brown T, et al. 2010. Atrazine induces complete feminization and chemical castration in male African clawed frogs (Xenopus laevis). Proceedings of the National Academy of Sciences of the United States of America 107(10): 4612-4617.

Iavicoli I, Fontana L, Bergamaschi A. 2009. The effects of metals as endocrine disruptors. Journal of Toxicology and Environmental Health Part B, Critical Reviews 12(3): 206-23.

INSERM (Institut national de la santé et de la recherche médicale). 2006. Collective Expert Report: Glycol ethers: New toxicological data.

Kato S, Fujii-Kuriyama Y, Ohtake F. 2007. A new signaling pathway of dioxin receptor ligands through targeted protein degradation. Alternatives to Animal Testing and Experimentation 14(special issue): 487-494.

Kitamura S, Suzuki T, Ohta S, Fujimoto N. 2003. Antiandrogenic activity and metabolism of the organophosphorus pesticide fenthion and related compounds. Environmental Health Perspectives 111(4):503-8.

Kitamura S, Sugihara K, Fujimoto N, Yamazaki, T. 2011. Organophosphates as Endocrine Disruptors. Anticholinesterase pesticides: metabolism, neurotoxicity, and epidemiology (eds T. Satoh and R. C. Gupta), John Wiley & Sons, Inc., Hoboken, NJ, USA.

Lacasaña M, López-Flores I, Rodríguez-Barranco M, Aguilar-Garduño C, Blanco-Muñoz J, Pérez-Méndez O et al. 2010. Association between organophosphate pesticides exposure and thyroid hormones in floriculture workers. Toxicology and Applied Pharmacology 243(1):19-26.

Laks DR. 2010. Luteinizing hormone provides a causal mechanism for mercury associated disease. Medical Hypotheses 74(4): 698-701.

Liao C, Kannan K. 2011. Widespread occurrence of bisphenol A in paper and paper products: implications for human exposure. Environ Sci. Technol. 45(21): 9372-9.

Lilienthal H, Hack A, Roth-Härer A, Grande SW, Talsness CE. 2006. Effects of developmental exposure to 2,2',4,4',5-pentabromodiphenyl ether (PBDE-99) on sex steroids, sexual development, and sexually dimorphic behavior in rats. Environmental Health Perspectives 114(2): 194-201.

Main KM, Kiviranta H, Virtanen HE, Sundqvist E, Tuomisto JT, Tuomisto J, Vartiainen T, Skakkebaek NE, Toppari J. 2007. Flame retardants in placenta and breast milk and cryptorchidism in newborn boys. Environmental Health Perspectives 115(10): 1519-26.

MDH (Minnesota Department of Health). 2006. Consumer Factsheet on: Dioxins. Minnesota Department of Health. October 2006.
http://www.health.state.mn.us/divs/eh/risk/chemhazards/dioxins.html

Meeker JD, Ferguson KK. 2011. Relationship between urinary phthalate and bisphenol A concentrations and serum thyroid measures in U.S. adults and adolescents from the National Health and Nutrition Examination Survey (NHANES) 2007-2008. Environmental Health Perspectives 119(10): 1396-402.

Mocarelli P, Gerthoux PM, Needham LL, Patterson DG Jr, Limonta G, Falbo R, et al. 2011. Perinatal exposure to low doses of dioxin can permanently impair human semen quality. Environmental Health Perspectives 119(5): 713-718.

Nagano K, Nakayama E, Oobayashi H, Nishizawa T, Okuda H, Yamazaki K. 1984. Experimental studies on toxicity of ethylene glycol alkyl ethers in Japan. Environmental Health Perspectives 57:75-84.

Patisaul HB, Roberts SC, Mabrey N, McCaffrey KA, Gear RB, Braun J, Belcher SM, Stapleton HM. 2013. Accumulation and endocrine disrupting effects of the flame retardant mixture firemaster® 550 in rats: an exploratory assessment. Journal of Biochemical and Molecular Toxicology 27(2): 124-36.

Post GB, Cohn PD, Cooper KR. 2012. Perfluorooctanoic acid (PFOA), an emerging drinking water contaminant: a critical review of recent literature. Environmental Research 116(24): 93-117.

Richburg JH, Nañez A, Gao H. 1999. Participation of the fas-signaling system in the initiation of germ cell apoptosis in young rat testes after exposure to mono-(2-ethylhexyl) phthalate. Toxicology and Applied Pharmacology 160(3): 271-8.

Rogers JA, Metz L, Yong VW. 2013. Review: endocrine disrupting chemicals and immune responses: a focus on bisphenol-A and its potential mechanisms. Molecular Immunology 53(4): 421-30.

Rossi-George A, Virgolini MB, Weston D, Cory-Slechta DA. 2009. Alterations in glucocorticoid negative feedback following maternal Pb, prenatal stress and the combination: a potential biological unifying mechanism for their corresponding disease profiles. Toxicology and Applied Pharmacology 234(1): 117-27.

Rubin BS. 2011. Bisphenol a: an endocrine disruptor with widespread exposure and multiple effects. The Journal of Steroid Biochemistry and Molecular Biology 127(1-2): 27-34.

Soldin OP, Braverman LE, Lamm SH. 2001. Perchlorate clinical pharmacology and human health: a review. Therapeutic Drug Monitoring 23(4): 316-31. Review.

Stanko JP, Enoch RR, Rayner JL, Davis CC, Wolf DC, Malarkey DE, Fenton SE. 2010. Effects of prenatal exposure to a low dose atrazine metabolite mixture on pubertal timing and prostate development of male Long-Evans rats. Reproductive Toxicology 30(4): 540-9.

Tonacchera M, Pinchera A, Dimida A, Ferrarini E, Agretti P, Vitti P et al. 2004. Relative potencies and additivity of perchlorate, thiocyanate, nitrate, and iodide on the inhibition of radioactive iodide uptake by the human sodium iodide symporter. Thyroid: Official Journal of the American Thyroid Association 14(12): 1012-9.

Walter H. Watson, James D. Yager. 2007. Arsenic: extension of its endocrine disruption potential to interference with estrogen receptor-mediated signaling. Toxicological Sciences 98(1): 1-4.

Wolff J. 1998. Perchlorate and the thyroid gland. Pharmacology Review 50(1): 89-105.

Wolstenholme JT, Rissman EF, Connelly JJ. 2011. The role of bisphenol A in shaping the brain, epigenome and behavior. Hormones and Behavior 59(3): 296-305.

Ya Wen Chen, Ching Yao Yang, Chun Fa Huang, Dong Zong Hung, Yuk Man Leung, Shing Hwa Liu. 2009. Heavy metals, islet function and diabetes development. Islets 1(3): 169-176.

Yamano T, Noda T, Shimizu M, Morita S, Nagahama M. 1993. Effects of diethylene glycol monomethyl ether on pregnancy and postnatal development in rats. Archives of Environmental Contamination and Toxicology 24(2): 228-35.

Zhu X, Kusaka Y, Sato K, Zhang Q. 2000. The endocrine disruptive effects of mercury. Environmental Health and Preventative Medicine 4(4): 174-83

Zota AR, Park JS, Wang Y, Petreas M, Zoeller RT, Woodruff TJ. 2011. Polybrominated diphenyl ethers, hydroxylated polybrominated diphenyl ethers, and measures of thyroid function in second trimester pregnant women in California. Environmental Science & Technology 45(18): 7896–7905.

http://home.earthlink.net/~joannefstruve/_wsn/page2.html

http://whole9life.com/2012/09/digestive-enzymes-101/

How Your Thyroid Works, 4th edition, by H. Jack Baskin, M.D. Adams Press, Chicago IL, 1995.

The Harvard Medical School Guide to Overcoming Thyroid Problems by Jeffrey R. Garber, M.D. with Sandra Sardella White, McGraw-Hill, New York 2005.

The Thyroid Gland: A Book for Thyroid Patients, by Joel I. Hamburger, M.D. Michael M. Kaplan, M.D. (self-published) Southfield, Michigan, 1991.

The Thyroid Sourcebook by M. Sara Rosenthal with a foreword by Robert Volpe, M.D., Lowell House, Los Angeles 1998.

Could It Be My Thyroid? The Complete Guide to the Causes, Symptoms, Diagnosis, and Treatments of Thyroid Problems (Foreword by George H.W. Bush) by Sheldon Rubenfeld, M.D. The Thyroid Society for Education and Research, Houston, Texas, 1996, 2002, 2003.

The Thyroid Book A Book for Patients by Martin I. Surks, M.D. (self-published) 1993, 1999.

Your Thyroid: A Home Reference, 4th edition, by Lawrence C. Wood, M.D., David S. Cooper, M.D., and E. Chester Ridgway, M.D. Ballantine Books, New York, NY, 2006.

http://thyroidpharmacist.com/articles/top-6-thyroid-tests

1. Katie J. Astell, Michael L. Mathai, Andrew J. McAinch, Christos G. Stathis, Xiao Q. Su. A pilot study investigating the effect of Caralluma fimbriata extract on the risk factors of metabolic syndrome in overweight and obese subjects: a randomised controlled clinical trial. Biomedical and Lifestyle Diseases (BioLED) Unit, College of Health and Biomedicine, Victoria University, Melbourne, Victoria 3021, Australia.

2. Niedzielin, K., Kordecki, H.,

http://journals.lww.com/eurojgh/Abstract/2001/10000/A_controlled,_double_blind,_randomized_study_on.4.aspx

3. M. Million, et al. Obesity-associated gut microbiota is enriched in Lactobacillus reuteri and depleted in Bifidobacterium animalis and Methanobrevibacter smithii. International Journal of Obesity (2012) 36, 817–825; doi:10.1038/ijo.2011.153; published online 9 August 2011

4. Rastmanesh R., et al. High polyphenol, low probiotic diet for weight loss because of intestinal microbiota interaction. Chemico-Biological InteractionsPublished 15 October 2010.

5. Thielecke F, et al. Epigallocatechin-3-gallate and postprandial fat oxidation in overweight/obese male volunteers: a pilot study Eur J Clin Nutr. 2010 Jul;64(7):704-13. doi: 10.1038/ejcn.2010.47.

6. Wang H., Effects of catechin enriched green tea on body composition. Obesity (Silver Spring). 2010 Apr;18(4):773-9. doi: 10.1038/oby.2009.256.

7. Bitange Nipa Tochi, Zhang Wang, Shi - Ying Xu and Wenbin Zhang, 2008. Therapeutic Application of Pineapple Protease (Bromelain): A Review. Pakistan Journal of Nutrition, 7: 513-520.

8. Date K, Satoh A, Iida K, Ogawa H. Pancreatic α-Amylase Controls Glucose Assimilation by Duodenal Retrieval through N-Glycan-specific Binding, Endocytosis, and Degradation. J Biol Chem. 2015 May 28. pii: jbc.M114.594937.

9.Perano SJ,Couper JJ,Horowitz M, Martin AJ, Kritas S, Sullivan T, Rayner CK. Pancreatic enzyme supplementation improves the incretin hormone response and attenuates postprandial glycemia in adolescents with cystic fibrosis: a randomized crossover trial.J Clin Endocrinol Metab. 2014 Jul;99(7):2486-93. doi: 10.1210/jc.2013-4417. Epub 2014 Mar 26.

◦ACAM (Amer. College for the advancement of medicine) http://www.acam.org/

◦APMA (Amer. Preventive Med. Assoc) http://www.apma.net/practitioners.htm

◦AHMA (Amer. Holistic Med Assoc) http://www.holisticmedicine.org/index.html

◦ABOUT.COM has 'Top Doc" listing http://thyroid.about.com/library/weekly/bldoc1.htm

◦and others like: ◦http://www.sonic.net/~nexus/listdocs.html

http://dujs.dartmouth.edu/fall-2010/the-physiology-of-stress-cortisol-and-the-hypothalamic-pituitary-adrenal-axis

(2) http://qjmed.oxfordjournals.org/content/93/6/323

(3) http://www.jbc.org/content/239/5/1299.full.pdf

(4) http://www.sciencedirect.com/science/article/pii/0009898181903533

(5) http://patient.info/doctor/pituitary-function-tests

1.J Clin Invest. 49;855-804, Braverman, L E.

2.Am J Physiol 1990;258:E715-E720, Pilo, A et al.

3.Clin Endocrinol (Oxf) 2002; 57:577-585, Saravana et al.

4.www.british-thyroid-association.org/armour.htm

5.Thyroid 13; 3-126, Balock, Z.

6.J Clinic Endo Metab 90; 5483-5488,Wartofsky, L.

7.Thyroid 2003; 13:3-126, Baloch Z, et al.

8.J Clinic Endo Metab 2005; 90: 5483-5488, Wartofsky, L et al.

9.Thyroid vol 22, No 12, 2012, Clinical Prac Guidelines.

10. J Clin Endo Metab 90; 5483-5488, Wartofsky,L

11. Thyroid 13;3-126, Baloch, Z.

12. Arch Intern Med 1981; 141: 873-875

13. Am J Med 1985:79; 271-276, Stryker T D, et al.

14. Endocrin Prac 2006; 12:572, Abdullatif H D, et al,

15. Public Health Nutrition 2007; 70:1606-1611.

16. Am J Physiol 90; 290-291, Boothby W M.

17. Thyroid 2001 Mar; 11 (3); 249-55.

18. J Clin Invest 1970; 49:855-864, Braverman L E et al.

19. NEJM 1999; 340: 424-429, Bunevicius R.

20. Int J of Neuropsychopharmacology 2000, June 3 (2): 167-174, Bunevicious R.

21. J Clin Endocrinol Metab 2003, 88(10), 4543-50, Walsh J P et al.

22. J Clin Endocrinol Metab 2006, 91:2592-2599, Grozinski- Glasberg, S.

23. Thyroid 2001 Mar, 11(3): 249-55, Padberg S.

24. Clin Endocrinol (Oxf) 72;709-715, Celi P S.

25. Intern Med 2000; 170: 19996, 2003, Bolk, N.

26. J Clin Endocrin Metab 2009; 94: 3905-3912, Bach-Huynh, T G.

27. Endocrin Prac 2003; 9: 363-369, Clarke, C D.

28. Clin Endocrin 1999;50:149-155, Pop V J.

29. Am J Clin Nutr 2008; 87:370-378, Raymon M P.

30. NEJM 2011; 364:1820-1931.

http://www.dana.org/Publications/ReportDetails.aspx?id=44163

The American Institute for Cancer Research. The New American Plate: A timely approach to eating for healthy life and healthy weight.

Fung, T. T. et al. Association between dietary patterns and plasma biomarkers of obesity and cardiovascular disease risk. American

Journal of Clinical Nutrition, January 2001. 73:61–67.

Centers for Disease Control. Overweight. April 2006. http://www.cdc.gov/nchs/fastats/overwt.htm

Alliance for a Healthier Generation. Alliance for a Healthier Generation Clinton Foundation and American Heart Association and Industry Leaders Set Healthy School Beverage Guidelines for US Schools. May 2006.

US Department of Agriculture. How much food from the meat and bans group is needed daily? http://www.mypyramid.gov/pyramid/meat_amount.aspx

Ogden, CL et al. High Body Mass Index for Age Among US Children and Adolescents, 2003-2006. Journal of the American Medical Association. 299(20):2401-2405. May 2008. http://jama.amaassn.org/cgi/content/short/299/20/2401

Higdon J, Delage B, Williams D, et al: Cruciferous vegetables and human cancer risk: epidemiologic evidence and mechanistic basis. Pharmacol Res 2007;55:224–236.

Wu QJ, Yang Y, Vogtmann E, et al: Cruciferous vegetables intake and the risk of colorectal cancer: a meta-analysis of observational studies. Ann Oncol 2012.

Liu X, Lv K: Cruciferous vegetables intake is inversely associated with risk of breast cancer: A meta-analysis. Breast 2012.

Liu B, Mao Q, Lin Y, et al: The association of cruciferous vegetables intake and risk of bladder cancer: a meta-analysis. World JUrol 2012.

Liu B, Mao Q, Cao M, et al: Cruciferous vegetables intake and risk of prostate cancer: a meta-analysis. Int J Urol 2012;19:134–141.

Lam TK, Gallicchio L, Lindsley K, et al: Cruciferous vegetable consumption and lung cancer risk: a systematic review. Cancer Epidemiol Biomarkers Prev 2009;18:184–195.

Bosetti C, Negri E, Kolonel L, et al: A pooled analysis of case-control studies of thyroid cancer. VII. Cruciferous and other vegetables (International). Cancer Causes Control 2002;13:765–775.

Dal Maso L, Bosetti C, La Vecchia C, et al: Risk factors for thyroid cancer: an epidemiological review focused on nutritional factors. Cancer Causes Control 2009;20:75–86.

Phytochemicals and Other Dietary Factors 2nd edition: Thieme; 2013

Krajcovicova-Kudlackova M, Buckova K, Klimes I, et al: Iodine deficiency in vegetarians and vegans. Ann Nutr Metab 2003; 47:183–185.

Leung AM, Lamar A, He X, et al: Iodine status and thyroid function of Boston-area vegetarians and vegans. J Clin Endocrinol Metab 2011;96:E1303–1307.

Office of Dietary Supplements, National Institutes of Health. Dietary Supplement Fact Sheet: Iodine.

Tonstad S, Nathan E, Oda K, et al: Vegan diets and hypothyroidism. Nutrients 2013;5:4642–4652.

McMillan M, Spinks EA, Fenwick GR: Preliminary observations on the effect of dietary brussels sprouts on thyroid function. Hum Toxicol 1986;5:15–19.

Chu M, Seltzer TF: Myxedema coma induced by ingestion of raw bok choy. N Engl J Med 2010;362:1945–1946.

Zhang X, Shu XO, Xiang YB, et al: Cruciferous vegetable consumption is associated with a reduced risk of total and cardiovascular disease mortality. Am J Clin Nutr 2011;94:240–246.

Fenwick GR, Heaney RK, Mullin WJ. Glucosinolates and their breakdown products in food and food plants. Crit Rev Food Sci Nutr. 1983;18(2):123–201

Chu M, Seltzer TF. Myxedema coma induced by ingestion of raw bok choy. N Engl J Med. 2010;362(20):1945–1946.

http://www.mercola.com/Downloads/bonus/dangers-of-nonstick-cookware/report.aspx

Takahashi Y, Kipnis DM, Daughaday WH Growth hormone secretion during sleep. J Clin Invest 1968;47:2079–2090.

Weitzman E. D., Fukushima D, Nogeire C, Roffwarg H, Gallagher T. F., Hellman L. Twenty-four hour pattern of the episodic secretion of cortisol in normal subjects. J Clin Endocriol Metab 1971;33:14–22.

Flegal, K. M. et al. Prevalence and Trends in Obesity Among US Adults, 1999–2008 JAMA. 2010;303(3):235–241.

Interviews with Melanie Polk, registered dietitian and director of nutrition education for the American Institute of Cancer Research

Interview with Marion Nestle, Marion Nestle, PhD, MPH, Chair of the Department of Nutrition and Food Studies at New York University

Interview with Barbara Gollman, registered dietitian and spokesperson for the American Dietetic Association

Nestle, M. and M. F. Jacobson. Halting the obesity epidemic: A public health policy approach. Public Health Reports, January/February 2000. 115:12–24.

http://www.nationofchange.org/ultimate-paradox-us-overfed-andmalnourished-nation-1372077901

http://www.aloeit.com/human-engine-our-bodies-health/

http://www.webmd.com/a-to-z-guides/hypothyroidism-topic-overview

http://www.mayoclinic.org/diseases-conditions/hypothyroidism/basics/symptoms/con-20021179

http://www.webmd.com/a-to-z-guides/hypothyroidism-topic-overview

http://hypothyroidmom.com/300-hypothyroidism-symptoms-yesreally/

http://www.womentowomen.com/thyroid-health/hypothyroidsymptoms-2/

http://www.medicinenet.com/hypothyroidism_symptoms/views.htm

http://www.stopthethyroidmadness.com/long-and-pathetic/

Mazokopakis EE, Starakis IK, Papadomanolaki MG, Batistakis AG, Papadakis JA. Changes of bone mineral density in pre-menopausal women with differentiated thyroid cancer receiving L-thyroxine suppressive therapy. Curr Med Res Opin. 2006;22:1369–73. [PubMed]

2. Mandel SJ, Brent GA, Larsen PR. Levothyroxine therapy in patients with thyroid disease. Ann Intern Med. 1993;119:492–502. [PubMed]

3. Singh N, Singh PN, Hershman JM. Effect of calcium carbonate on the absorption of levothyroxine . JAMA. 2000;283:2822–5. [PubMed]

4. Singh N, Weisler SL, Hershman JM. The acute effect of calcium carbonate on the intestinal absorption of levothyroxine. Thyroid. 2001; 11:967–71. [PubMed]

5. Neafsey PJ. Levothyroxine and calcium interaction: timing is everything. Home Health Nurse. 2004; 22:338–9. [PubMed]

6. Mazokopakis EE. Counseling patients receiving levothyroxine

(L-T4) and calcium carbonate. Mil Med. 2006;171:vii,1094.

[PubMed]

[No authors listed]. Iodine. Monograph. Altern Med Rev 2010; 15(3):273–278.

Leung AM and Braverman LE. Iodine-induced thyroid dysfunction. Curr Opin Endocrinol Diabetes Obes 2012; 19(5): 414–419.

Brahmbhatt SR et al. Thyroid ultrasound is the best prevalence indicator for assessment of iodine deficiency disorders: a study in rural/tribal schoolchildren from Gujarat (Western India). European Journal of Endocrinology 2000;143:37–46.

Brahmbhatt SR et al. Study of biochemical prevalence indicators for the assessment of iodine deficiency disorders in adults at field conditions in Gujarat (India). Asia Pacific J Clin Nutr 2001; 10(1):51–57.

Kris-Etherton PM, et al. Polyunsaturated fatty acids in the food chain in the United States. Am J Clin Nutr 2000; 71(1):179S-188S.

Carrington J. Using hormones to heal traumatic brain injuries. [Internet]. Available at: http://www.lef.org/magazine/mag2012/jan2012_Using-Hormones-Heal-Traumatic-Brain-Injuries_01.htm.

Kresser C. How too much Omega-6 and not enough Omega-3 is making us sick. [Internet]. Available at: http://chriskresser.com/how-too-much-omega-6-and-not-enough-omega-3-is-making-us-sick.

•Panda S, et al. Withania somnifera and Bauhinia purpurea in the regulation of circulating thyroid hormone concentrations in female mice. Journal Ethnopharmacology 1999; 67(2):233-9.

Panda S, et al. Changes in thyroid hormone concentrations after administration of ashwaganda root extract to adult male mice. Journal of Pharmacology 1998; 50:1065-1068.

Kalani A, et al. Ashwagandha root in the treatment of non-classical adrenal hyperplasia. BMJ Case Reports 2012; 10(1136).

Agrawal P, et al. Randomized placebo-controlled, single blind trial of holy basil leaves in patients with noninsulin-dependent diabetes mellitus. Int J Clin Pharmacol Ther 1996; 34(9):406-9.

Gholap S, et al. Hypoglycaemic effects of some plant extracts are possibly mediated through inhibition in corticosteroid concentration. Pharmazie 2004; 59 (11):876-8.

Khan V, et al. A pharmacological appraisal of medicinal plants with antidiabetic potential. J Pharm Bioallied Sci 2012; 4(1):27-42.

Norman A. From vitamin D to hormone D: fundamentals of the vitamin D endocrine system essential for good health. Am J Clin Nutr August 2008; 88(2):491S-499S

http://www.mayoclinic.org/healthy-lifestyle/fitness/in-depth/exercise/art-20048389?pg=2

http://healingthebody.ca/coconut-sugar-a-low-gi-sugar-rich-in-amino-acids-and-b-vitamins/

http://info.visiblebody.com/endocrine-system-hypothalamus-and-pituitary

http://www.progressivehealth.com/low-levels-t3-t4.htm

http://www.fluoridealert.org/wp-content/uploads/merck-1968.pdf

http://fluoridealert.org/issues/health/thyroid/

Recipes (as in the measured list of ingredients) and very short directions on how to combine those ingredients are not protected under the various forms of copyright law. This is because they fall under the designation of being the steps in a procedure and they're explicitly excluded from copyright. Countries which are signatories to either the Berne convention or the Buenos Aires convention use the same basic standard to determine what is and isn't copyrighted although there are small local variations. However, the exclusion on procedures is not a local variation. What can be copyrighted are the more complex directions that usually accompany the list of ingredients in modern recipes. As long as you rewrite any directions to be in your own words you've followed the law. Cooking something from a recipe recorded by someone else and selling it is legal.

www.ingramcontent.com/pod-product-compliance
Lightning Source LLC
Chambersburg PA
CBHW070224190526
45169CB00001B/72